MW01485566

"Martina Williams and Kyle Wehrend's book on reparent

book on Internal Family Systems (IFS) and its amazing skills to help us to find the power and ability to bring ourselves back into a secure attachment within, reparenting ourselves with the love and healing we may not have received as children. It helps us to remember that it is never too late to have a happy childhood."

—**Kay Gardner, MS, LCPC**, IFS Institute Senior Lead Trainer

"Martina and Kyle offer a warm, practical, and neuroscience-informed approach to reparenting from within. Using real examples from their own lives and decades of clinical experience, they walk you through everything you need to know about IFS to begin working with your own parts."

—**Risa Adams, MD**, IFS Institute Co-Lead Trainer and coauthor of *It Doesn't Have to Be This Way*

"Martina and Kyle are beautiful and gentle souls who have created a heartfelt companion for your IFS journey in their book, *An IFS Reparenting Workbook*. The book is solid with both dependable and concise guidance, offering clear language and key exercises to support readers on their IFS journey. Navigating one's internal world can be both confusing and overwhelming, especially when working through childhood trauma. This workbook not only presents clear guidance and experiential exercises, but Martina and Kyle also accompany you on your journey through their shared encouragement, normalization of important moments, and the realizations they offer from their own healing experiences."

—**Chris Burris, LMFT**, IFS Institute Senior Lead Trainer and author of *Creating Healing Circles*

"This is the IFS workbook you've been waiting for! Kyle and Martina offer a clear and personal introduction to the IFS model that is filled with practical exercises, supportive meditations, and individual stories that make the work come alive. Information about attachment and neuroscience will help you to deepen understanding of how your parts are formed, burdened, and ultimately healed."

—**Elizabeth Parsons, MD, CCFP**, Certified IFS Therapist, and coauthor of *It Doesn't Have to Be This Way*

"Martina and Kyle draw on both their clinical experience and their own healing journeys to show that struggles like anxiety, perfectionism, and low self-esteem are not flaws, but the burdens of wounded parts longing for care. With warmth and clarity, they offer readers a way to build relationships with those parts and bring the healing presence of Self."

—**Richard C. Schwartz, PhD**, founder of Internal Family Systems (IFS)

"This workbook guides readers through the application of IFS in a clear, accessible way, with experiential exercises and real-life examples that bring the model to life. If you're looking to integrate parts work into your daily life and to tend to the parts of you that need healing, this is a resource you'll return to again and again."

—**Leslie Petruk, MA, LCMHC-S**, IFS Institute Lead Trainer and director of the Stone Center for Counseling and Leadership

AN **IFS** REPARENTING WORKBOOK

**Internal Family Systems
Skills to Heal
Childhood Trauma,
Nurture Secure Attachments
& Embrace Radical
Self-Acceptance**

Martina Williams, LCMHC
Kyle Wehrend, LICSW

New Harbinger Publications, Inc.

Publisher's Note

NEW HARBINGER PUBLICATIONS is a registered trademark of New Harbinger Publications, Inc.

New Harbinger Publications is an employee-owned company.

Copyright © 2026 by Martina Williams and Kyle Wehrend
New Harbinger Publications, Inc.
5720 Shattuck Avenue
Oakland, CA 94609
www.newharbinger.com

Cover design by Amy Shoup

Acquired by Jed Bickman

Edited by Joyce Wu

Library of Congress Cataloging-in-Publication Data on file

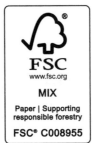

Printed in the United States of America

28   27   26

10   9   8   7   6   5   4   3   2   1   First Printing

Martina—*To my husband, George,*
who teaches me the true essence of love
and embraces my parts with endless warmth and unwavering acceptance.

Kyle—*To my daughter, Aza,*
for teaching me how to be a papa;
to my son, Endri, for teaching me how to be a child again;
and to my wife, Ryan, for always being my secure base.

Contents

Acknowledgments

We would like to express our deepest gratitude to our teachers and mentors, Richard Schwartz, Deb Dana, Stephen Porges, Jon Kabat-Zinn, and Kristin Neff. We also want to extend our deepest gratitude to Ralph De La Rosa, Susan McConnell, Chris Burris, Jenna Riemersma, Risa Adams, Leslie Petruk, and Elizabeth Parsons for their support of our workbook. We would like to thank our developmental editor, Madison Davis, acquisitions editor, Jed Bickman, and our copyeditor, Joyce Wu. Last, but definitely not least, we would like to acknowledge all of our clients over the years who have taught us more about our own internal systems than they will ever know: Our heartfelt gratitude for sharing your lives with us.

In celebration of our dear friend and colleague, Ralph De La Rosa, 1976-2025.
A tireless advocate for compassion and social justice, Ralph made the world feel safer for all of us impacted by trauma and suffering. Their life and work is a shining example of the power of Self-led healing.

Foreword

This foreword was meant to be written by Ralph De La Rosa. Ralph was deeply admired, and their presence and contributions left a meaningful mark on the Internal Family Systems community. I am honored to carry their light forward here, with profound gratitude for the path they walked and the wisdom they shared. It is an unexpected privilege to write in their place, and I do so with deep respect and reverence.

This workbook is a gift. Not just because it distills the transformative wisdom of Internal Family Systems, but because Martina and Kyle bring it to life with such authenticity, warmth, and clarity. Drawing from the rich soil of attachment theory, polyvagal theory, mindfulness, and somatic practices, they have created a guided journey that is both transformative and deeply empowering. Their words gently illuminate how we can turn inward with compassion, connect with our managers, firefighters, and exiles, and begin to lead our systems—and our relationships—from Self.

What truly sets this work apart is how personal it is. Martina and Kyle are not speaking at us; they are walking alongside us. Through real-life stories, including their own, they model what it means to speak on behalf of our parts rather than from them, and how to approach repair—not only within ourselves but with the people we love—with integrity and grace. This is more than a workbook. It is an invitation into a new way of relating—with ourselves, others, and the world around us. Whether you're brand new to IFS or a seasoned traveler on this inner path, you'll find support, insight, and genuine connection in these pages. May this book carry forward the spirit of those who've guided us—past and present—and may it help you find deeper harmony within and without. Your inner journey awaits!

With warmth and gratitude,

Jenna

Jenna Riemersma, LPC

Introduction

Hello and welcome! We're glad you're here.

If you're reading this right now, it's entirely possible that you have asked some variation of the following questions:

"Can Internal Family Systems help me?"

"Is Internal Family Systems for doing therapy with families?"

"What's the deal with this 'parts' stuff?"

"WTF is 'IFS'?!"

We'll address all these questions and more in this workbook. Internal Family Systems (IFS) offers a beautifully simple framework that for some can be intuitive and easy to grasp. Yet, in our own experiences with the IFS model, having a helping hand along the way can dramatically improve how well you can incorporate the model into your daily life. Whether you're just starting out or already well on the way in your IFS journey, our goal is to offer a welcoming and straightforward approach to support you in your own unique process.

In our humble opinions (and with over four decades of experience between us), the IFS model is one of the most effective psychotherapy modalities out there at the moment. Until fairly recently, the major focus of other modalities has been to focus on what's wrong or "disordered" with our clients. Popular modalities, such as cognitive behavioral therapy (CBT) or dialectical behavior therapy (DBT), posit that to be healthy and high-functioning, we need to learn how to control our thoughts, feelings, and behaviors by overriding or replacing "negative" or "irrational" thoughts with rational ones. Or that the best someone can hope for in therapy is to learn how to cope with the challenges of daily life through techniques and skills that can result in incremental progress.

While these approaches are certainly effective in providing measurable results and have supported people in making incremental improvements in how they respond to their daily stressors, as clinicians (and human beings), we'd like to think we can do better than that. As opposed to offering only gradual progress, IFS can promote *transformational* change. Instead of centering the work around our challenges and limitations, IFS offers a message of hope: *You have a limitless resource for healing already present inside of you.* This resource, present within each of us, is a wise, compassionate "Self" capable of gently reparenting and healing our childhood wounds.

Self comes preloaded in everyone with all the love, compassion, and strength you'll ever need to take care of yourself and feel connected to those around you.

For this reason, we view IFS as more than just a psychotherapy model. Unlike approaches that confine you to a rigid set of beliefs and principles, IFS is open, flexible, and adaptable to your unique individuality. Reparenting from Self empowers you to become your own nurturing caregiver and frees you up to rely less on external sources for validation and well-being. This paradigm shift in the IFS model encourages a profound U-turn (or, as we prefer to call it, a "you-turn"), showing you how to look inside to tap into your innate wisdom for guidance and support.

Many common challenges (like anxiety, procrastination, perfectionism, low self-esteem, loneliness, and lack of confidence) often arise from childhood attachment wounds that we have suffered and continue to carry. From the perspective of the IFS model, these struggles are not seen as disorders, character flaws, or personal shortcomings. Instead, they are understood as manifestations of injured, young, vulnerable parts within us. By learning to work with these parts, IFS can help in numerous ways, perhaps most importantly by addressing and healing childhood wounds and traumas at the root level.

The model is wonderfully moldable and comprehensive in its ability to address a wide array of issues and challenges. Overall, it can teach you how to manage stress and navigate life transitions more effectively. It can enhance emotional regulation by giving you a better understanding of your emotions and how to express them in beneficial ways, and it can strengthen your communication skills for more meaningful relationships.

If you, like most of us, experience internal conflict, IFS can help bring harmony to your inner world, easing tension and supporting emotional well-being. If external conflict feels challenging, IFS can also guide the internal parts of you toward healthier, more effective ways of navigating those difficult situations.

Behaviorally, it can help you overcome challenges such as procrastination, perfectionism, substance abuse, and disordered eating. Finally, many find internal clarity, which allows for discovering and pursuing their life purpose with a sense of direction and fulfillment.

This may seem like a tall order to fill! We get it. We wouldn't have believed IFS could help with such an array of symptoms and issues either if we had not experienced it ourselves or in our clinical work with countless clients. But it is truly a flexible and comprehensive way of looking at ourselves and the world around us.

If the inner wisdom of Self can help us in so many ways, what separates us from our ability to tap into it? The answer lies in the IFS concept that we all have "parts," or aspects of ourselves that step in to respond to whatever life throws at us, and some of which prevent us from accessing our inherent wisdom. We hear this use of the "part" concept in our language: A part of me wants to go out with my friends tonight, but another part wants to stay in and relax.

Most of our parts develop when we are young. They arise as coping strategies and behaviors in response to our biological need to survive and find ways to stay connected to our caregiver(s). For example, if you had an angry caregiver who went into rages, you may have developed a people-pleaser part who worked hard to avoid triggering your caregiver. This behavior can carry over into your adult relationships where you might find yourself working hard to avoid your supervisor's or partner's wrath.

These parts can get frozen in time, causing you to react from whatever age the part formed, as with the people-pleasing example above. You may think you are reacting from your adult self, when in fact your reaction is most often from a younger part ranging in emotional age from infancy through young adulthood. What this means is that when you become highly reactive to a situation, it may be because you are experiencing the world through the eyes of a younger version of you.

If any of this feels a bit confusing, don't worry; we'll get into all of this in more detail in the chapters to come. For now, we just encourage you to go into this workbook with an open mind, some curiosity, and a healthy bit of skepticism. After all, we want you to take your time with what we're suggesting here. Try these techniques and perspectives out and decide what works for you. We hope that through the information and experiences offered in this workbook, you will begin to see yourself with more warmth and compassion, learn to appreciate the wonders of your own vast and complex inner world, and begin to tap into the limitless internal resources you have for healing and Self-guided growth.

If you feel lost along the way, get off track, or even feel like giving up, we want you to know: We understand. There's no judgment here. The beauty of having all of this information in one place is that you can always come back to it again and again. In fact, we recommend that! Regardless of when and how you decide to utilize this workbook, we'll be here for you whenever you want to return.

How to Use This Book

We and our clients have benefited greatly from the approaches we are going to share with you in this book and in the online materials at the publisher's website, http://www.newharbinger. com/55909, which includes expanded examples, case studies, and bonus exercises. Here are some gentle suggestions for how you might get the most out of them going forward.

Take Your Time

Remember the old saying about the journey being more important than the destination? That wisdom applies here too. This is not a book to race through like a spy novel. Instead, treat it like a leisurely walk in the park on a sunny Sunday, where you savor every moment. As you read, you'll develop observation skills, self-awareness, insights, and a stronger sense of Self, all of which are essential for healing your internal wounds.

As IFS senior trainer Chris Burris is fond of saying, "Slow is fast." Taking your time leads to faster, better results in the long run. Let that be your mantra if you begin to feel a sense of urgency about getting to the end.

Do the Exercises!

This is an experiential journey. To get the full benefit of this book, we recommend doing all the exercises and meditations provided. While it might be tempting to just read and understand the content intellectually, remember that learning to ride a bike requires actually getting on the bike. Similarly, IFS is not a cognitive process. Learning is more like a staircase than an elevator. It's not possible to get to the top of the staircase without walking up each step.

To truly benefit from this book and the IFS model, you need to actively participate in the exercises. These exercises are essential building blocks for understanding and using the complete model. Don't shortchange yourself. A few dedicated minutes now will pay off in the long run, we promise!

Enlist a Buddy

Do you thrive on motivation and accountability when you have a buddy by your side? Is everything more fun when it's shared? If that sounds like you, why not team up with a friend who's eager to dive into this model alongside you?

Set Aside Time

In the whirlwind of your busy life, it is common to juggle countless responsibilities. It's easy to prioritize the needs of others over your own. However, for true, lasting change, it's important to create time to focus on your growth and development. Imagine setting aside special time just for you—like making a date with yourself. Mark it on your calendar. These dates don't need to be long; start with just thirty minutes once a week. Think of the time dedicated to this workbook as a precious investment in yourself. Remember, consistency is the key to success. The more you tune in to your inner world and follow the steps in this model, the more skilled you'll become. It's just like mastering any new skill: Practice, practice, practice!

Set an Intention

Consider setting an intention for what you would like to accomplish as you make your way through this workbook. It could be something specific, such as "I treat myself better after making a mistake," or broader, like "I feel more confident in my interactions with others." Having a specific reason for engaging in this work can go a long way toward keeping you focused if you get lost or lose motivation.

To learn about intentions and how to set them, go to the bonus content on the publisher's website for this book, http://www.newharbinger.com/55909.

Keep a Parts Journal

We highly recommend starting a "parts journal" to keep track of and "map out" your parts and how they relate to each other and to Self. It can be as simple as writing down each internal part you come across with some simple descriptors. (For example, problem solver part, tension in my forehead, says, "How can we fix this ASAP!" They show up in response to other people telling me about their problems.) A more elaborate approach can be creating a family tree or genogram visually depicting how parts are connected and how they interact. Some folks like using art to depict how they experience their parts. Whatever works for you. As long as you find it helpful as a way to depict externally what is going on for you internally.

Take Self-Compassion Breaks

And last, but definitely not least: go easy on yourself! Doing something new is not easy and can often feel unfamiliar or even uncomfortable at times. This is what learning is all about, and learning takes time and effort. If, while working on this workbook, you catch yourself in moments of frustration, discomfort, or confusion, we encourage you to stop, take a pause, gently place your hand on your chest, and breathe slowly and deeply. You might even say something to yourself like *This is what learning feels like—that's all this is*, or *This is really hard for me right now*.

After taking a self-compassion break, if you decide to pick the workbook back up and try again, great! If not, also great! There's no judgment here and there's no one way to go about using this workbook. Make it your journey and try to be kind to yourself in the process.

Each chapter will build on the previous chapter to give you a solid understanding of the IFS model, so we recommend working through this book sequentially. You will learn about your inner system of *protective* and *wounded* parts and how to tap into your inner resource of Self to help them heal. This will all make sense later. Just know that we structured the book to be as gentle and intentional as possible to support your journey of inner healing.

When to Seek Professional Help

While we believe that you can make progress solely through the use of this introductory workbook, we do feel strongly that to fully absorb the depth of the IFS model, you can benefit greatly from having the support of an IFS therapist. Many readers of this book may find it is most helpful as a support while working with a practitioner.

Doing this kind of internal work can stir up some strong feelings, emotions, or sensations. If at any point traumatic memories emerge or your symptoms worsen or feel like more than you can handle individually, please seek help from a trained professional. If you are interested, you can find available IFS-trained therapists at http://www.IFS-institute.com.

Who Are We?

We are two clinically licensed therapists with decades of experience helping clients.

Not only are we clinicians, but as people, we have experienced our own traumas, struggles, and setbacks. We are both actively engaged in our own inner work with IFS therapists. We speak not only from our experience using the IFS model with our clients but also from our own lived experiences of healing through this model.

I (Martina) am a trauma recovery therapist who began as a hospice counselor in 1999. Several years prior, I started traditional talk therapy. It provided insight and understanding. I then began EMDR (eye movement desensitization reprocessing), which was powerful in addressing single-trauma incidents like recovering from an abusive boyfriend. But it didn't heal my deeper child-hood wounds, which kept showing up in my romantic relationships. I continued to unconsciously attract and be attracted to emotionally unavailable partners. It felt like something was wrong with me. Why couldn't I change my behavioral patterns when I intellectually understood the problem? I didn't realize I suffered from childhood attachment trauma until I discovered IFS. I learned to build relationships with my younger wounded parts and began reparenting them. It transformed my life both personally and professionally. Since 2011, I've used IFS as my primary therapy method, witnessing profound, life-changing healing in countless clients. It truly facili-tates healing at the root level.

I (Kyle) am a clinical social worker with over fifteen years of experience. Before becoming a therapist, I worked in medical and school settings with adults and teenagers whose lives were heavily impacted by trauma. It wasn't until the birth of my daughter during the COVID-19 pan-demic, when I experienced an intense and prolonged bout of paternal postpartum depression, that I began to come to terms with my own trauma history. Through my work in session with my IFS therapist, I gradually came to understand the correlation between things that happened to me as a child and how I was reacting to my daughter. The IFS model helped me to identify the root cause of my troubling or problematic reactions to things in the present and provided me with a gentle and compassionate framework for how to heal from these painful and scary childhood experiences.

We've worked with many people who have faced immense suffering in their lives, whether it be childhood trauma, emotional neglect, or attachment injuries, and we've found the IFS model consistently provides the support and stable base that many of them were looking for. No matter what your background, we feel confident that IFS can help improve your life.

Okay, here we go. We're with you each step of the way.

CHAPTER 1

Adaptive Strategies and Behaviors:
How Parts Are Formed

The basic structure of the IFS model is pretty simple. There is *Self* and there are *parts*. Of course, there's more to it than that (otherwise, you wouldn't need a whole workbook to make sense of it). But for now, let's just start with the basic concepts and go from there.

What Is Self?

Okay, so what is this thing called *Self*? Well, it can be difficult to put into words, but here we go: Self is a limitless source of comfort, love, support, and strength that we are all born with. Each of us has a true Self deep within our core. We were born with Self and it cannot be harmed or damaged. It is whole. It is this Self within each of us that can step in and reparent us, be the loving, wise, and responsible adult we needed when we were younger. Why the capital *S*? The capital *S* is just a way to distinguish it from the more common use of the word "self," which tends to view a person as one unified personality, such as "she didn't seem like her*self* when she acted like that."

The Self doesn't inherently possess a personality, role, or agenda. Being agenda-less, the Self is often most accessible when we stop striving for something or trying to control our environment. We recognize it when we allow ourselves to simply settle into being present with whatever is. Some call this a state of flow.

We're not suggesting that the Self is only accessible when you're doing nothing. Rather, it's about being aware of your motivation. If your actions are driven by an agenda, fear, or avoidance, you're not embodying the Self. On the other hand, if you approach an action with a sense of calm, clarity, and openness, you're more aligned with what the IFS model refers to as being Self-led. Let us give you an example.

I (Kyle) was attempting to write this section explaining the Self but was frustrated by my inability to put into words something so familiar to me. When interacting with clients, I find it relatively easy to transition into a warm, nonjudgmental, compassionate, and open presence in my sessions. But I was having a hard time translating that into something I thought you as the reader might understand. I was feeling stuck.

Once I realized what was happening, I slowed down and gently checked in with myself to notice my thoughts and feelings. I heard one voice telling me to get the wording "just right," another voice worrying I would never get it "right," and yet another voice expressing frustration with having to deal with the stress of work. That frustration felt like increasing pressure in my body and I could feel my body getting hotter as my heart rate increased. Soon, I began to distract myself by looking up random facts online, checking my email over and over, or going to the kitchen to look for more snacks. I was looking for any way to escape the inner struggle and avoid working on this workbook!

By slowing down for a few minutes, I recognized the voices as different "parts" of myself, which shifted my perspective and provided clarity. I paused to appreciate that these parts were each trying to help me deal with the discomfort being caused by work. With this understanding, I viewed their efforts (the distraction, the frustration, the concern) with compassion. A warm feeling of calm settled over me and a burst of creativity filled my mind. I returned to writing with less inner conflict and more confidence, realizing that this section of the workbook didn't have to be perfect. By simply checking in with myself, I found it easier to write.

Can you identify with any aspects of Kyle's story? Take a moment to remember a situation when you faced a task and felt stressed, frustrated, or overwhelmed. How did you handle it? Did you start engaging in distracting behaviors like turning to your phone or the internet? Perhaps you went into overdrive and tried to just push through the discomfort? As you reflect, pay close attention to physical sensations in your body (e.g., tingling, heat, pressure) as well as your thoughts.

_____

_____

_____

_____

_____

_____

_____

If all this talk about the Self doesn't fully make sense, that's okay. Stick with us and try some of the exercises we outline in this workbook. We're confident you'll start noticing how Self appears in your life and begin to experience what we mean. As mentioned, the Self isn't something you can understand purely intellectually—it's a state of being. This might seem too vague for some of you, and that's okay. See if you can allow yourself to be comfortable with that uncertainty, just for now.

The Universality of "Self"

Religious and spiritual traditions offer diverse perspectives on the universal concept of a wise and compassionate core Self. While IFS doesn't align with any specific tradition, its idea of Self resonates widely. Some, but not all, are listed here. Mystical Christianity speaks of the "inner Christ" or "divine spark," reflecting God's essence within us. Jewish Kabbalah describes the "Neshama," a divine spark connecting us to God. Buddhism emphasizes "Buddha-nature," the potential for enlightenment embodying purity, wisdom, and compassion. Sufism refers to the *ruh* (spirit) or *qalb* (heart) as a divine presence guiding unity with God. These teachings collectively reveal the universal presence of a deeper, divine essence.

What Is Self to You?

Do you have spiritual beliefs that shape your understanding of a core Self? What qualities define it? Reflect on moments of full presence—deep conversations, flow states in work or exercise, or bursts of creativity. These effortless, doubt-free experiences may reveal a connection to your true Self.

Take a moment to reflect and write down examples from your life when you experienced something similar to the idea of "Self" we're describing. These moments could be significant, like the instant your newborn baby looked into your eyes or you felt the cool mist of a waterfall on your face. Or they might be smaller, everyday experiences, like catching the warm smile of a friendly stranger or watching a leaf dance in the sunlight.

As you reflect, take your time to truly revisit these moments. Imagine yourself there again and notice how they feel in your mind, your body, and the space around you in this moment. When you're ready, use the space below to jot down anything you'd like to capture from this exercise.

Self moments: _____

_____

_____

_____

_____

Qualities of Self

As he was beginning to develop the IFS model, originator Dr. Richard Schwartz began to notice specific qualities emerging in all of his clients. Dr. Schwartz identified eight qualities that start with the letter *c*: *calmness, curiosity, compassion, confidence, courage, creativity, clarity,* and *connectedness.* As it turns out, these qualities are also present in all of us.

If you revisit the section above about Kyle trying to write about the Self, you'll notice that once he was able to slow down and look inward, he gained perspective and *compassion* for himself, leading to a sense of *calm.* This inner shift sparked a burst of *creativity,* allowing Kyle to persist in his writing with greater patience and *confidence.*

You might be thinking, *Do I really possess all these qualities? I've never seen myself as calm or particularly confident.* That's okay. We will help you identify your own qualities of Self and learn to use them in your daily life. Let's start with an exercise to help you personalize this concept.

EXERCISE: Self Qualities

As you look at the illustration on the following page, take some time to describe what each of these words means to you. We recommend printing out the online PDF available at http://www.newharbinger.com/55909 or writing your definitions in your journal. Your understanding of what these qualities are and how they show up for you may change as you get to know yourself better, so we recommend coming back to this section again and again to update and evolve your understanding of how these qualities of Self show up in your life. For example, *courage* doesn't mean the absence of fear, but rather acting despite it, even when the outcome is uncertain or difficult. It involves taking steps forward with openness and vulnerability, knowing that growth and meaningful change often require stepping outside of your comfort zone. *Confidence* might be defined as a grounded trust in your ability to handle challenges, navigate uncertainty, and act successfully, based on self-awareness, past experiences, and a belief in your capacity to grow and adapt.

Next, can you think of examples of when one of these qualities showed up in your life or when you may have wished they had been able to show up? Write your answers on your printout or in your journal.

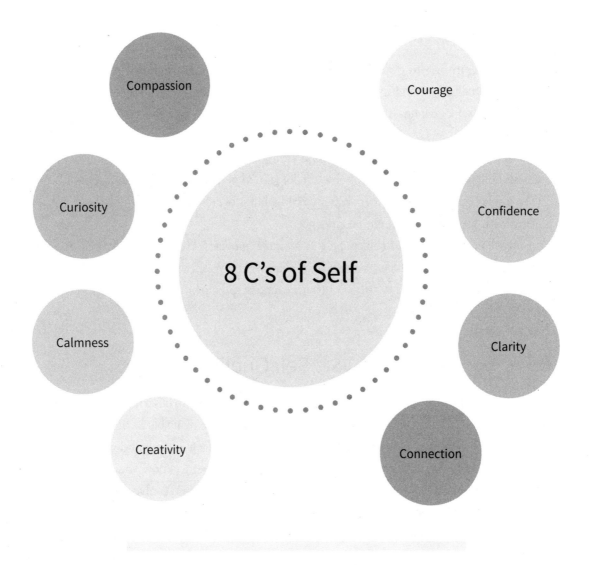

We encourage you to consider *making this a daily practice*. It can be as easy as pausing for a few minutes each day to review moments where you felt "in Self," a state of being where you embody these Self qualities and relate to yourself and others with a sense of balance, understanding, and care. And if some days you can't find any examples, that's okay. As you begin to heal from old wounds, you will naturally feel in Self, more in touch with your core of *compassion*, more often. Being in Self means that the Self is leading.

Now that you have a rough idea of what Self is, let's take a look at the other IFS concept: parts! We bet you can remember a time when you were having a conversation with someone and you felt super defensive or vulnerable. These are parts, not Self.

What Are Parts?

So, when we talk about this idea of *parts*, what do we mean?

Well, think about your own life. You might already be experiencing this concept and not realize it. For example, if you go to a restaurant and you're trying to figure out what you want to order, you might say, "Well, part of me wants to get the french fries, but another part of me wants to order the salad." Or if you argue with a family member, a partner, or a friend, you might say, "Part of me realizes that they were right, but part of me wants to stay angry at them."

In most cases, you might just make a decision and move on with your life. What IFS encourages us to do is slow down and get curious about what each one of those parts is communicating. Going back to the restaurant example, if you give attention to the part of you that wants the french fries, they might be saying something like "Mmmmm, french fries are delicious. They make me feel good when I eat them. I'm tired of having to watch what I eat all the time."

Now, let's get curious about the part of you that wants to order salad. That part might be saying something harsh and shaming, like "If you eat french fries, you'll get fat!" or something cautionary like "Everyone will judge you if you order fries instead of salad." Maybe this part is concerned about your health and reminds you there's a history of high cholesterol in your family. They equate fried foods with cholesterol and say something like "French fries are bad for you. Salad is the healthy choice."

None of these parts are inherently wrong or bad. Each have their reasons for wanting you to choose one option over the other, and those reasons are rooted in your life experiences. For example, the part of you craving french fries might want you to feel good in the moment because they remember how eating fries brought comfort in the past. If you dig deeper, this part might also carry a desire to rebel against restrictive eating rules imposed on you as a child, or they might hold memories of using comfort food as your only source of self-soothing when no one else was there for you.

On the other hand, the part that wants you to choose the salad may be motivated by an awareness of societal norms and the messages you've internalized about health and appearance. It feels like they're looking out for you. Going even further back, this part may have emerged to protect you from being criticized about your weight by a caregiver during childhood. Both parts are acting from a place of care shaped by your personal history.

As you can see in this example, there's more going on inside than we might initially be aware of. The examples above speak to a kind of inner back-and-forth that we all go through, sometimes daily. In IFS, this internal struggle is referred to as a *polarization*, or any point of ongoing tension between two or more internal parts.

The Internal Tug of War

The concept of polarization is fundamental to understanding how your parts interact and impact your daily functioning. Polarizations typically occur between parts that disagree. For example, a productivity part might be polarized with a "binge TV" part. One part wants to get things done and the other part wants to relax. Polarizations can feel like an inner tug-of-war, pulling you in different directions.

Have you ever felt this internal tug-of-war unfolding in your mind? That's completely natural! What might seem like random thoughts are often different parts of you communicating. These internal exchanges can range from major decisions, like a career change or ending a relationship, to minor choices, like whether to take a lunch break or picking a shirt color. Such interactions happen constantly and profoundly shape how we navigate the world. (For an internal tug-of-war exercise, see the bonus content at http://www.newharbinger.com/55909.)

Noticing skeptical parts showing up? That's great—we welcome them! We have them too. Fun fact: "Skeptical" comes from the Greek root *skeptikós,* meaning "thoughtful and inquiring."

• *Am I Losing It?*

When I (Martina) got sick at the age of thirty-four, I dropped twenty-five pounds in a month. I had to temporarily close my private practice as a spiritual counselor, and I started experiencing almost daily panic attacks. It was a frightening time. One day, while driving, I felt like five different voices were yelling at me in my head. I pulled to the side of the road to center myself and try to sort out the voices. One said, "You've got cancer they haven't found!" Another said, "You have no money, you're going to lose your apartment!" And yet another said, "Your new husband is going to leave you!" and "You're going to die!"

I was terrified I was losing my mind! I called a psychologist friend who reassured me that my experience was common with severe anxiety. While that was comforting, the experience made me keenly aware that I had different voices in my head. That didn't seem "normal" to me at the time. So, I bought a book on CBT and tried to consciously change these voices, with some success. It wasn't until years later, when I discovered IFS therapy, that I accepted that those voices were natural. They were actually parts of me giving me warning messages and wanting me to take action. I started getting to know these parts rather than try to change them.

Just like Martina, the conversations in your head are parts giving you messages. So, let's explore what's going on inside of you!

EXERCISE: What Are Your Parts Saying?

Begin by taking a long, deep inhalation through your nose and slowly exhale through your mouth. Repeat this a few more times. Next, either close your eyes or soften your gaze by letting your eyes go out of focus.

Take a moment to reflect on your day so far and record your responses in your journal:

- Do you notice any thoughts?

- Perhaps you have an ongoing mental laundry list? "Remember to buy eggs and pay the water bill." How do these reminders make you feel? Do you notice any sensations, like an urge to move or take action?

- Perhaps you are replaying a conversation over and over while criticizing yourself. *Why did you say that? You sounded stupid. You should have said x, y, z instead!* How do these messages make you feel? Are there any emotions present?

- Did you notice anxious messages: *How am I going to meet that deadline?* or *I am dreading the family reunion.* How does your body react to these messages? Tightness? Increased heart rate?

- Perhaps you have depressing thoughts such as *It's hopeless. I'll never meet anyone!* or *If they really knew me, they wouldn't like me.* Is there sadness present? Or do you feel like curling up in a ball?

Now let's put this into the context of parts. Did you notice anything similar to the examples we provided? If so, then it's probably a part. If not, did you experience some kind of pushback against the idea of internal parts? If so, that, too, was probably a part. As you consider this idea of internal parts, does it change how you view the thoughts circulating in your head?

Multiplicity of Mind

Psychologist Richard Schwartz, the founder of IFS, views "voices" or "parts" as natural and universal. He discovered something powerful through years of clinical work: Each of us is made up of many "parts" or subpersonalities, each with their own thoughts, feelings, and purpose (1997). These parts aren't a sign that there is something wrong—they're a natural part of being human.

Think about feeling torn between two choices. Or catching yourself in an inner debate. That's the mind's multiplicity in action. Schwartz's approach helps us make sense of these everyday inner conflicts, not as flaws, but as conversations or behaviors happening within a larger, dynamic inner system.

Traditional psychology often sees the mind as one single ego in control. Schwartz offers a refreshing and compassionate alternative—one that embraces our inner complexity rather than labeling it as a disorder. In Martina's above example, she thought something was wrong with her, that she had developed some mental disorder.

Not only is multiplicity of mind a universal experience, it's innate. We are born with parts and in their natural state, they are free and all get along wonderfully. If you've ever had the pleasure of staring into an infant's eyes while they are looking back at you, you might get a sense of this inner harmony. There's no indication of self-doubt or shame or judgment. Just a pure sense of wonder and curiosity.

Parts Are Internal Resources

Parts are internal resources that help us function and thrive in our daily lives. Many of our parts go unnoticed because what they are doing, their "role," is not causing any kind of disruption in our life at the moment. In fact, many of our parts are important to our daily functioning. As adults, we need parts that care about meeting our financial responsibilities and paying our bills. Some part of us needs to care about our emotional responsibilities to those we love. We need to get to work on time. We need to remember *how* to get to work. You get the point.

Our internal parts often believe they are helping, but they can sometimes misfire because they interpret situations through a lens shaped by past experiences. These parts rely on coping strategies that were unconsciously formed in childhood, influenced by our family environment. If our needs weren't met, if we felt unsafe around caregivers, or if we experienced significant challenges or trauma, these parts developed survival mechanisms to protect us. Many of us have experienced adverse childhood experiences (ACEs). In fact, "during 2011–2020, nearly two thirds of U.S. adults reported at least one ACE, and approximately one in six U.S. adults reported four or more ACEs" (Swedo et al. 2023, 73). It is crucial to understand this concept and its potential impact on your development and the development of your parts.

ACEs

ACEs can be considered a variety of difficult or traumatic events that occurred before the age of eighteen. Some examples might be experiencing or witnessing violence or abuse, growing up in an environment that lacked consistent access to basic needs like food, water, and shelter, or the separation from caregivers as a result of divorce, death, or incarceration. Multiple large-scale research studies were conducted in the last thirty years regarding ACEs. The UNC Frank Porter Graham Childhood Development Institute reports that "ACEs often have lasting, negative effects on health and well-being, as well as life opportunities such as education and labor market opportunity... The accumulation of (or exposure to) multiple ACEs, rather than experiencing any single type of ACE, is most predictive of negative outcomes" (Gitterman et al. 2024, 2).

If you are interested in taking a free ACEs test, go to this link: https://www.npr.org/sections/health-shots/2015/03/02/387007941/take-the-ace-quiz-and-learn-what-it-does-and-doesnt-mean.

While not everyone has had a traumatic childhood, most of us have had distressing or impactful experiences. Your early childhood experiences affect the development of your brain and can have lasting impacts on your physical, emotional, and mental health. These experiences can even impact you later in life in ways that may seem unrelated or surprising, such as limiting your ability to learn, preventing you from making a living, and even contributing to chronic health issues.

EXERCISE: Trace Your ACEs

Looking at individual experiences may not seem that impactful, but when you plot them across a timeline, you can get a sense of the cumulative effect of the events over the course of your life. All of these events left their mark on you. Understanding this impact will help you as we get further into the model.

We have provided a timeline graph with examples of significant childhood experiences, both adverse and impactful. The graph is divided into age ranges for easy reference. You may have encountered challenging experiences at different ages. Everyone's timeline is unique.

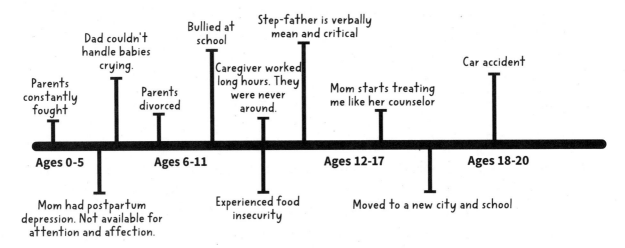

Adverse Childhood Experiences

Now it's your turn. Take a moment and begin to reflect on what challenges and impactful experiences you went through in childhood. Keep in mind that some events may not seem impactful looking back. After all, we know only our own lived experience, so whatever we went through may feel "normal" to us. We invite you to include any potentially impactful events, no matter how big or small they might seem. Feel free to discuss with safe family, friends, and others who were around during your childhood to get their perspectives as well. When you're ready, plot them along the timeline in the appropriate age categories. Don't worry if you can't remember the exact ages.

Childhood Adverse or Impactful Experiences

Ages 0-5

Ages 6-11

Ages 12-17

Ages 18-20

How was that for you? What's it like to see these experiences on a timeline? Can you get a sense of what the cumulative effect might have been for you?

_____

_____

_____

When you had these hard experiences, was there anyone there to help you get through it, to make it better, to help you make sense of what happened? If so, who was that person and how did they support you?

_____

_____

_____

_____

If not, you may have received "insufficient emotional attunement." It is only with "sufficient attunement", that we overcome the painful impact of these challenges (more on this in chapter 2). So, if you were on your own, we have a pretty good idea of how you coped. You likely used your internal resources, your natural gifts, and your abilities to meet the challenge. In IFS language, a *part* steps forward and takes on a *role* to help you. This is where *protective* parts come in.

Protective Parts

Our parts are clever and resourceful, using their natural gifts and abilities to create coping strategies that helped us navigate challenging situations *at that time*. These strategies become their roles. For example, a part that is naturally independent, imaginative, and content playing alone might take on the role of self-sufficiency if a caregiver was frequently unavailable.

If a caregiver was highly critical, it may have felt like rejection, leaving us with deep pain and a sense of shame. In response, a part that naturally pays attention to fine details might adopt the role of striving for perfection to avoid criticism. Similarly, a naturally supportive, cheerleader-like part might become overwhelmed by frequent criticism and take on the role of being self-critical, hoping to preempt external criticism.

Our parts didn't form in response to just our home environments—they also adapted to situations at school, with peers, or in other social settings. For example, a part might have stepped in to lead a group activity if no one else took charge, or they might have mimicked the behavior of popular kids if we struggled to fit in. In cases of social anxiety, a part may have coped by withdrawing and trying to stay unnoticed. Childhood social situations present a wide range of challenges, and our parts are shaped by how we respond to them.

Exiles

In IFS, our wounded parts are called *exiles*. They are the parts that carry vulnerability, pain, and shame. Have you ever noticed how uncomfortable it can be to feel rejected, hopeless, or embarrassed? It's painful. And humans dislike pain. We will often do our best to not feel any pain. Wouldn't it make sense that if we experienced something deeply painful, whether it was physical, emotional, or mental pain, we might try and push it away or *exile* the part carrying the pain?

Exiled parts are typically created in childhood, often as a result of feeling disconnected from our caregiver(s) or experiencing distressing, painful, or traumatic events. For example, if your caregiver couldn't handle your expressing your emotions, you might have been told, "You're too sensitive—toughen up, don't be a crybaby!" A part of you internalizes this message, believing it to be true. This part may conclude that there's something wrong with you and that you're unlovable. So, the next time you are given that message (and there's always a next time), another part (a protective part) steps in to hide your sensitivity by choking back tears and pretending like nothing is wrong.

Imagine your caregiver exploding in rage when you made a mistake, yelling, "You're a piece of crap! Can't you do anything right?" Over time you begin to believe them. Their criticism becomes your truth. To cope, a protective part numbs you, but deep down, an exiled part still believes you're unworthy of love. Though untrue, these beliefs make sense given your experience.

All Parts Are Welcome

If we are all born with a core Self, what goes wrong? First, we need a caregiver to help uncover and nurture the gifts and qualities of this Self. Second, every childhood involves challenges. What might seem trivial or silly as an adult could have felt overwhelming or impossible as a child. Even with "ideal caregivers," it's impossible for them to provide perfect emotional support all the time. So, what's the solution?

Self is the healing force that can address our childhood wounds. Even if your caregiver could suddenly offer the emotional support you needed, they wouldn't be able to heal your deepest parts because they missed that crucial window. Healing must come from within. The good news is that you can tap into the beautiful qualities and endless resources of your Self, which we'll explore more deeply later on.

We love the analogy of parts being like the weather. The Self is like the sun, always there shining in the sky. But parts can come in and cause turbulent or unpleasant weather, making it hard to feel the presence of Self guiding us. When we get to know our parts and build a relationship with them, we can ultimately trust the sun will shine again and provide us with warmth and nurturing.

Protectors don't intend to bring bad weather into your life. Quite the opposite. Their intentions are always positive, even if their actions sometimes lead to unintended consequences. While it may be tempting to rely on labels like "good parts" and "bad parts," an important aspect of the IFS model is its mantra: All parts are welcome. It may be tempting to assume that we should just try and get rid of parts or ignore them, especially ones that seem to be causing us trouble, but that would only make matters worse. The more we try to push away parts of ourselves, the more internal tension and struggle we create. This effort to hold back these parts is unlikely to benefit us in the long run.

It's also not possible to get rid of parts. That would be like trying to get rid of your arm. It's a part of you. After all, these parts keep us functioning. As we noted, they handle our daily responsibilities. They make sure we pay our bills, feed our children, and get our work done. We need our parts to help us navigate our world, our environments (beginning with our home environment), then school and among friends.

A judgment-free attitude will greatly help you to get to know your parts—build a relationship with them and care for them—to bring healing and lasting change. And here is where your loving, *compassionate* Self within can *reparent* these parts. It is your loving, *compassionate* Self who can witness, hear, and understand your wounded inner children. Instead of saying "I hate that part!" or "I wish that part of me would stop, go away, or relax!" we encourage you to ask yourself this question: *Given that none of my parts are bad, why would they show up the way they do?*

The saying "the squeaky wheel gets the grease" applies to our internal parts as well. The more intense a part is, the more likely they are to grab your attention and prompt a response to their perceived threats. Right now, you have a complex system of internal parts focused solely on ensuring your survival. Their dedication to this purpose can be quite comforting.

We encourage you to approach your parts gently and patiently, helping them recognize that you've survived the original threat they reacted to. Since then, you've grown and experienced much more. As they begin to understand this, they may be more willing to step back, allowing your current self—armed with life experience and support—to take charge moving forward.

Do you have parts that you dislike or think are bad? Take a moment to write down several aspects of yourself that you may dislike or wish were different.

_____

_____

_____

_____

Now go back through that list and see if you can identify what each aspect, or part, might be trying to protect you from.

_____

_____

_____

_____

_____

_____

_____

Trailheads

In the IFS model, a *trailhead* is any sign that helps you notice an internal part, like muscle tension, a change in tone of voice, or a mood shift. These signals serve as entry points for exploring and understanding our inner parts, often appearing as thoughts, feelings, sensations, memories, or behaviors. Anything that prompts you to pause and look inward is considered a trailhead.

EXERCISE: What Are Your Trailheads?

Let's work to identify some of your trailheads. Think about an upsetting event. Describe the event:

_____

_____

_____

_____

_____

_____

_____

_____

Now, play the memory back on repeat for a few moments and pay attention to how it felt emotionally and physically *at that time*.

_____

_____

_____

_____

These feelings and sensations are your trailheads!

You can do this exercise as many times as you like to identify more trailheads. (Visit the website at http://www.newharbinger.com/55909 for a printable copy.)

Conclusion

In this chapter, we introduced the core Self as a limitless resource of inner wisdom and positive qualities. We explored how childhood challenges can leave emotional wounds, leading parts of us to emerge as protective mechanisms. These parts shield us from further pain and help us cope. We also discussed how the core Self can guide and support the healing of these wounded parts.

In chapter 2, we'll explore attachment theory, signs of caregiver misattunement, and how they shape our attachment style. These insights reveal how, driven by the need to stay connected to caregivers, our parts developed strategies to meet our needs. Understanding these patterns is key to recognizing how they still influence us today, helping us separate from past experiences and move toward healing and self-compassion.

CHAPTER **2**

In a Lonely World, IFS Can Help

We've all felt the sting of loneliness at one time or another. It's part of the human condition. One way we might define loneliness is through a subjective lens, as a discrepancy between our felt sense of social connection and our desired level of social connection (Peplau and Perlman 1982).

In our current environment, many of us find it difficult to know how or where to connect with others in a meaningful way. The technologies that promise ease and convenience often result in a dramatic reduction of face-to-face, in-person interaction with other human beings.

There has also been a decline in community and civic engagement over the decades. Robert D. Putnam's book *Bowling Alone: The Collapse and Revival of American Community* documents the decline in what he refers to as "social capital" in the U.S., illustrating how people have become less involved in community organizations, less likely to join clubs, and less engaged in communal activities (2000). The COVID-19 pandemic made this issue even worse, resulting in many people experiencing more intense or prolonged bouts of isolation with little to no relief. According to a Meta-Gallup report (2023), nearly a quarter of the global population feels "very" or "fairly lonely." The report comes from research done on connection and loneliness from 142 countries.

Furthermore, many of us live in echo chambers, meaning that we seek out and listen to only those who already share our point of view. We seem to have lost the ability to listen and connect, especially across social, familial, economic, and political divides. As a result, there is an increasing number of groups who feel unseen, receiving the message that they don't matter. This is concerning because, as humans, we all have an inherent need to be known, seen, valued, and understood. As individuals and groups, we frequently feel excluded or are made to feel different. This amplifies the lack of social trust we witness all around us. How many of us can genuinely look into the eyes of a stranger without feeling a little scared at times?

Reflection

Take a few minutes to pause and reflect on how loneliness may have been present at times in your own life. Write the responses to the following prompts in your journal:

- What times in your life have you felt lonely?

- Have you experienced frequent feelings of loneliness?

- Do you sometimes feel lonely even when you are around family, friends, or work associates?

Do you use social media to connect with others? How does social media impact your feelings of connection? How does it impact your feelings of loneliness or isolation?

What are we to do with increasing levels of isolation and lack of access to genuine connection? We believe a significant part of the answer lies within each of us, in the dimension of *intra*-personal connection (i.e., connection to self). In other words, there are parts of us who never experienced the attunement, connection, and attachment we needed from our caregiver(s). The scars and wounds of childhood left us lonely for genuine connection. Fortunately, we can start healing loneliness by making connections within.

Healing Internal Loneliness

IFS provides a way to heal our deep, internal loneliness, enabling us to improve the external, interpersonal connections in all our relationships. And for some of us, healing the loneliness within allows us to create safe relationships with others for the first time. As your authors, we both have known the struggles of chronic loneliness. Through discovering and embarking on personal and professional journeys with IFS, we are actively healing significant aspects of our childhood pain. We are excited to share this transformational model and support you in your journey. We will begin by sharing a bit of our own stories.

• *Martina's Story*

Martina discovered IFS during a difficult period marked by back surgery, constant pain, a heavy workload, her mother's worsening dementia, and the end of a relationship. Despite professional success and strong friendships, Martina struggled with chronic loneliness and longed for an intimate partner. Her relationships often ended in rejection because she became overly anxious and too eager to please, suppressing her true self to avoid abandonment.

Martina's childhood abandonment after her parents' divorce drove her to unconsciously seek validation from emotionally unavailable men. Working with a therapist who introduced her to the IFS model, she realized a wounded inner child (exile) shaped her romantic choices. By nurturing this part, Martina healed, learned self-love, and no longer sought redemption through a partner.

As she healed, her chronic loneliness dissipated, and she approached dating with a sense of wholeness. In time, she met and married an emotionally present man who accepts her for who she is. Through the journey of IFS and love, Martina continues to heal and grow, embracing her true self and writing her own love story.

Pause and take a moment to think about your relationship history. This can be with family members, friends, or romantic partners. In what ways have you struggled? Do you notice any recurring patterns?

• *Kyle's Story*

Starting around adolescence, Kyle began to feel a hollowness inside that he was sure could be filled only by the attention of a romantic partner. He longed to find someone he thought could fill that hollowness, but felt crippled by insecurity and fear of rejection. He spent much of his teenage years into early adulthood flooded with anxiety and self-doubt and would experience periods of depression. After his first girlfriend broke up with him, he experienced an intense bout of depression and began to rely heavily on alcohol to self-soothe and to help manage his anxiety.

While enrolled in grad school for social work, Kyle's clinical supervisor suggested he begin individual therapy and linked him up with his first therapist. He instantly clicked with this therapist and began experiencing improvements in the daily anxiety he was experiencing. He poured himself into learning more about coping skills and eventually started a mindfulness meditation practice. While he felt like he was getting to know himself better than ever before, he still relied heavily on alcohol to make him feel better and struggled to find romantic partners. And that hollow feeling still kept showing up.

At a psychotherapy conference in Washington, D.C., Kyle discovered the IFS model, which resonated deeply with him. Working with an IFS therapist, he explored the link between his loneliness and alcohol use in a compassionate, nonjudgmental way. This journey helped Kyle uncover childhood traumas still shaping his thoughts and behaviors. Using IFS, he learned to access his inner resources during moments of sadness, finding a sense of wholeness and connection.

Can you relate to Kyle's story? Take a moment to reflect on how you typically respond to discomfort. What do you do when feeling depressed, anxious, stressed, or lonely? Do you seek support from others or handle things alone? Do you use devices for distraction or prefer quiet time to process your emotions? There's no judgment—just curiosity about the behaviors you turn to during tough times and where they might have begun.

Follow the prompts below to explore your own behavior patterns:

Think of an uncomfortable situation, then write down what you notice: thoughts, feelings, physical sensations, and so forth.

_____

_____

_____

How do you typically respond? (Write down behaviors, statements, and activities that might occur in response to what is making you uncomfortable.)

_____

_____

_____

Feel free to repeat this exercise with as many examples as you like in your journal. The more attention you give to your habits and behaviors, the easier it will be to begin identifying internal parts later.

As we illustrated in our stories above, we believe an aspect of the answer to the loneliness epidemic lies within our childhood experiences. From the moment we are born, we leave the safe, protected space of the womb and enter the world with a need to "attach" to our caregiver(s). *Attachment* is a natural human survival instinct to connect with the people who take care of us. Attachment impacts how we move toward and away from our caregivers, as a baby and then as a toddler, and it shapes how we will behave in other relationships later in life, such as those with romantic partners and friends. This understanding of human development is rooted in what is known as *attachment theory*.

Attachment Theory

To highlight attachment's significance, consider the following: As mammals, we have basic survival needs: food, water, and shelter, to name a few. However, as human beings, we have an additional requirement that is just as important: emotional needs. When we are young, we are unable to meet these needs independently; we need caregivers. We are completely reliant on our caregiver(s) to read our emotional signals, ranging from distress to joy, and respond accordingly. If crying loudly resulted in our caregiver getting upset or distressed, or if our caregiver was unable or unwilling to respond to our cries, we may have learned to shut down, numb out, or find other ways of getting their attention, such as acting out.

Luckily for us, we don't have to learn how to connect to our caregiver(s) after we're born because we are naturally wired for attachment. As a result of this wiring, our early years are heavily influenced by the folks who take care of us and by their ability and willingness—or lack thereof—to respond to our needs. According to John Bowlby, the British developmental psychologist who originated attachment theory, if we receive the kind of attention from our caregiver(s) that results in our feeling seen, heard, and valued as a child, then we are more likely to move forward with a sense of security about ourselves and about the world around us (Holmes 2014).

Attachment Styles

Another attachment theorist, Mary Ainsworth, introduced the concept of *attachment styles*. The aforementioned attachment style would be referred to as *secure attachment*, meaning that there was a felt sense of security, safety, and consistency in how a child's caregiver(s) responded to the child's needs over time (Bretherton 1992).

Unfortunately, many people don't receive enough attunement from their caregivers. *Attunement* is the ability and willingness of a caregiver to be aware of and to respond to a child's needs. In other words, to *tune in* to us. Attunement is directly related to the quality of the bonds we make with our caregiver(s). *Misattunement* happens when the caregiver can't or won't meet the needs of the infant or child. This leads to *insecure attachment*, forcing us to develop coping strategies to survive and fulfill our needs.

Key Concepts

- Secure attachment—an internalized sense of safety, security, and *connectedness* in relationships

- Insecure attachment—an internalized sense of fear or uncertainty about relationships

- Attunement—a caregiver's ability to effectively respond to a child's physical and emotional needs

- Misattunement—a caregiver's inability or unwillingness to respond to a child's physical and/or emotional needs

Our early coping mechanisms shape what psychoanalyst John Bowlby calls our *internal working model*, a blueprint for understanding ourselves and others (Bowlby 1969, 1982). This model, crucial for survival in childhood, continues to guide our relationships into adulthood—whether at work, with family, or in love. When emotional needs go unmet in youth, forming secure bonds later can be difficult. However, recognizing these patterns allows us to build healthier connections.

Consider this list of signs that you may have experienced misattunement. Check which ones you experience in your daily life:

☐ Chronic feelings of emptiness

☐ Loneliness

☐ Unmet needs for love, acceptance, or approval

☐ Anxiety

☐ Anger or rage

☐ Self-criticism

☐ Lack of confidence

☐ Low self-esteem

☐ Lack of self-acceptance

☐ Despair

☐ Hopelessness

☐ Helplessness

☐ Depression

Self Can Heal Misattunement

If you recognize any of those signs of misattunement, you're not alone. Everyone can identify with the feeling of not being heard, seen, or understood, or not getting their needs met. As living beings, there's a difference between what we *want* and what we *need* to survive. Our wants can be as infinite as our imagination. But what we need to survive is very specific to each person. Unfortunately for us, since our nervous system does not decipher between real events and imagined events, the imagined list of things we want can get quite long and can cause quite a bit of emotional and physical turmoil.

The great news is that you don't have to stay stuck in an outdated internal working model. IFS offers a profound message of hope addressing the repercussions of childhood adversities and unmet needs. This evidence-based psychological approach directly engages with the aspects of your psyche that are impacted by misattunement and that continue to operate as though we are still trapped in those past experiences.

Our message isn't to "blame your caregiver(s)!" They were shaped by their own experiences, as were the generations before them. Caregivers can't give what they didn't receive, and it's impossible to meet every need of a growing child. Nor would doing so prepare them for the challenges of the real world. A certain level of adversity is essential for growth and resilience, but too much can leave lasting wounds.

The great news is that you can heal by tapping into Self—the part of you that is naturally *calm, compassionate, clear, creative, courageous, curious, confident,* and *connected.*

Imagine your Self possessing all these wonderful qualities, stepping in to reparent you by providing the love, attention, and care that your young parts didn't receive. It is a significant personal breakthrough to be able to help heal the parts of you that are still reacting to childhood experiences, to essentially enable you to reparent yourself. As Richard Schwartz (2021, 107) notes, "IFS can be seen as attachment theory taken inside, in the sense that the client's Self becomes the good attachment figure." And because IFS is in essence an attachment model, let's begin with helping you understand the four styles of attachment: secure, anxious, avoidant, and fearful-avoidant.

Secure Attachment

Imagine growing up in a warm, supportive environment with patient caregivers who provided comfort in tough times, encouraged exploration, nurtured your creativity, and supported your individuality. Expectations were clear and explained, with feedback given constructively and without fear or punishment. This ideal caregiver attunement fosters *secure attachment* through availability, accessibility, and consistent responsiveness.

Sounds pretty good right? Just to be clear, someone who exhibits this attachment style is not "better" than other people. This kind of attachment style is only a result of some pretty incredible attention provided by someone's caregiver(s) or individual work done by the person. It's literally like winning the caregiver lottery.

We didn't all experience secure attachment in childhood and so have been left with unmet developmental needs. To cope with this, we unconsciously formed strategies and behaviors to stay connected and attached to our caregiver(s). Remember, staying connected to our caregivers is a biological imperative; there is no shame in this. We had to find ways to survive. Problems arise when we carry childhood strategies into adulthood, as these approaches often no longer align with our current circumstances.

Identifying some of these behaviors and strategies—or insecure attachment styles—will help prepare you to understand and use the IFS model.

Insecure Attachment Styles

Three basic attachment styles arise from misattunement. We will help you understand them below.

Anxious (or Preoccupied) Attachment

Anxious attachment arises when caregivers are inconsistent in providing security, whether through emotional or physical availability or limiting independence. Those with this attachment style often struggle with low self-worth, fear of rejection or abandonment, and distress when separated from loved ones. They may also engage in people-pleasing behaviors to maintain relationships.

Avoidant (or Dismissive) Attachment

Avoidant attachment develops when a child is raised by an emotionally distant caregiver. In response, the child learns to suppress their emotional needs and rely solely on themselves. As adults, individuals with this attachment style tend to avoid emotional closeness. They often appear detached in relationships and typically experience low anxiety, even when intimacy is lacking.

Fearful-Avoidant (or Disorganized) Attachment

Fearful-avoidant attachment forms when a child experiences an abusive or unpredictable caregiver, creating confusion around safety and connection. As adults, they crave closeness but fear it, leading to high relationship anxiety and a push-pull dynamic, alternating between seeking intimacy and pushing it away, often marked by intense, conflicting emotions.

EXERCISE: What Is Your Attachment Style?

Check the following boxes you identify with the most.

Anxious Attachment/Preoccupied Attachment

☐ I worry when I am apart from my partner that they will become interested in someone else.

☐ I fear that, if my partner/friend got to know my true self, they would not like me.

☐ I get jealous/fearful when my partner/friend spends time with others.

☐ I get nervous if my partner seems preoccupied, distant, or unhappy.

☐ I get anxious if my partner/friend doesn't respond to my texts quickly.

☐ I had to find ways to soothe/comfort myself.

☐ I find ways to repeatedly ask for reassurance from my partner/friend: Are you mad at me? Did I do something wrong? Do you find me attractive?

☐ I feel preoccupied with my relationship. I think about it all the time.

Avoidant Attachment/Dismissive Avoidant

☐ I want to be close to my partner or have close friends, but intimacy feels too scary or almost claustrophobic.

☐ I want to spend time with my partner/friends, but always need to have an escape route or excuse to cancel plans if I need to.

☐ I long for a partner, but my freedom and independence are too important to me.

☐ It's hard for me to open up to my partner/friend.

☐ I feel uncomfortable being touched or physically affectionate.

☐ I dislike feeling pressured to open up.

☐ It's hard for me to accept criticism, even if given constructively.

☐ I distance myself from unpleasant emotions by choosing to turn my attention to hobbies or work.

Fearful-Avoidant Attachment/Disorganized Attachment

☐ I find it difficult to trust others.

☐ I have a hard time regulating my emotions.

☐ I have a negative view of others and/or myself.

☐ I may find myself anxious if my partner is unresponsive to my needs, but can feel claustrophobic if they get too close emotionally.

☐ I find myself spacing out, in another world.

☐ I have a hard time coping with stress.

☐ I crave attention, but don't know how to ask for it.

☐ If I get upset, I can shut down and be unable to communicate how I feel while simultaneously hoping my partner will read my mind and reach out.

Secure Attachment

- ☐ I feel comfortable relying on my partner/friends.

- ☐ I feel safe sharing my emotions and needs with my partner/friend.

- ☐ I am genuinely interested in my partner's/friends' hobbies or activities.

- ☐ I take the time to truly listen and understand my partner's/friends' fears and concerns.

- ☐ I feel comfortable providing and receiving consistent emotional support.

- ☐ I feel comfortable being myself around others.

- ☐ I feel comfortable spending time alone or with others.

- ☐ I feel capable of taking care of myself, and when I can't, I ask for help.

Whichever category has the most checks may be an indication of your attachment style(s). Keep in mind that many of us have more than one attachment style. It can be very situational. For example, we may exhibit characteristics of secure attachment with friends, but anxious attachment romantically.

To be clear: Our attachment patterns do not define us. They are a result of our inherent desire to survive the environment that we had no control over as a child. Take solace in the fact that these patterns of behaviors are flexible, which means that they can be adapted and modified to respond to your *present* experiences and to rely less on your *past* experiences.

You may be surprised at how far-reaching the impact of insecure attachment styles can be. It can affect our mental health, social interactions, self-perception, school and work performance.

As you read the following, take some time to consider how your attachment style(s) may be affecting your own life. For example, if you identify with the anxious attachment style, do you find yourself struggling with fear of abandonment and feelings of insecurity, constantly seeking reassurance and validation from your partner? Do you experience low self-esteem, lack of confidence, or anxiety? Perhaps these behaviors have negatively impacted your relationships with others, resulting in them pulling away from you.

If you identify with the avoidant attachment style, you may be prone to maintain emotional distance from others and struggle with intimacy, preferring self-reliance. Do you suppress emotions or have difficulty identifying or expressing your feelings? Do you have trouble trusting or relying on others? Do you avoid conflict with family and/or friends? Do you long for connection, but are scared to lose your independence?

If you can see yourself in the fearful-avoidant attachment style, it might mean you have high levels of anxiety and fear in relationships. Do you have a history of chaotic, unstable relationship patterns? Like people with avoidant attachment, you may desire closeness while also fearing it. Is emotional regulation challenging? Do you find yourself experiencing intense emotional reactions when interacting with others or experiencing difficulties in managing stress in interpersonal conflicts?

Protective Behaviors Connect to Parts

Whatever attachment style(s) you identified with most, it's not good or bad. If you have struggled with your attachment style, it's not your fault. It's also not your caregivers' fault. As a child, you were wired to seek connection with your caregiver. If they couldn't provide a secure attachment, you developed thoughts and behaviors to protect that bond. These responses, formed in early survival stages (e.g., food, comfort, shelter), were designed to keep you safe. As you grew, these protective behaviors became default reactions to similar threats.

To understand your parts better, think of these protective behaviors as ways your inner parts formed to maintain a connection with your caregiver(s). Insecure attachment often leads to common behaviors, which you can identify and name. For example, if you had a highly critical caregiver, you might have developed an inner critic to preemptively criticize yourself before they could. If you avoided conflict, you may have formed a people pleaser. If your caregiver was emotionally distant, you could have created a performer to seek attention. If emotions weren't allowed, you might have developed a masking part to hide your feelings.

It can be helpful to connect your behaviors to specific parts of you. In this way, you can begin to see the ways that you respond to things in your life as merely *a part* of you and not who you are all of the time. As you look at the list below, see if you identify with any of the behaviors that some of these common internal parts engage in. This preliminary work will make it easier when you get to the chapter where you start working with individual parts.

EXERCISE: What Behaviors Did You Develop?

To explore the behaviors you developed, find a quiet place where you can concentrate. Read the list of common behaviors that can form into parts as a result of insecure attachment. Put a check mark next to the ones that resonate with you.

☐ Perfectionist part: trying to be perfect or focused on imperfections or how things could be better

☐ Critical part: highly critical of others

☐ Inner-critic part: self-critical or focused on the ways that you're not doing something well

☐ Inner-judge part: judgmental toward self or others (i.e., focused on shoulds and should nots)

☐ Pleaser part: focused on pleasing others or being liked by others

☐ Fixer part: focused on "fixing" yourself

☐ Doer part: need to constantly be doing something or producing

☐ Approval-seeker part: seeking approval from others

☐ Masker part: feeling the need to hide or mask feelings

☐ Chameleon part: changing your personality according to whom you're around

☐ Controller part: focused on maintaining a sense of control

☐ Stonewaller part: blocking out others' access to your emotions (a.k.a. "stonewalling")

☐ Thinker/analytical part: prioritizing rational thoughts over emotions

☐ Planner part: always planning or fixated on future-oriented duties or activities

☐ Caretaker part: focused on other people's needs above your own

☐ List-maker part: focused on drafting never-ending to-do lists

Which behaviors or thoughts jump out at you (pick three to five)? Reflect on how each one shows up in your life.

_____

_____

_____

_____

_____

_____

_____

_____

_____

Are there any other thoughts or behaviors not on the list that you feel come from an insecure attachment with your caregiver(s)?

_____

_____

_____

_____

_____

Protective Thoughts Connect to Parts

Psychological models often emphasize changing thoughts and behaviors. For example, CBT encourages us to replace irrational thoughts with rational ones, while behavior modification therapy focuses on altering our behaviors. IFS takes a different approach. What may seem irrational from the outside makes complete sense from a parts perspective. Rather than trying to change the way our parts think and behave, an IFS approach focuses instead on understanding why our parts think and behave the way they do. These thoughts and behaviors are not random; they originate from different parts within us.

By connecting with our Self qualities, we then build relationships with our protective parts and learn how their behaviors aim to help us. As these parts come to trust the Self as a caretaker, they may let go of their old roles. Most protectors develop in childhood based on what we experience as children and these protectors' strategies can be updated as we grow and learn new ways to cope. For example, a perfectionist part might shift to striving for excellence, and a caregiver part may learn it's okay to prioritize self-care. This journey helps protectors release the burdens they've carried.

As you read this client story, can you start to identify behaviors and strategies that may be coming from one of Alex's young parts?

• *Alex's Story*

Alex came into therapy after his current partner threatened to break up with him, complaining that Alex was too emotionally distant. Alex said this was a familiar complaint from previous romantic partners and had contributed to multiple breakups in the past. He said he wanted to learn how to communicate his emotions better, but that he felt lost and unsure of where to start.

When asked about his upbringing, Alex stated he was raised in a two-parent household where his father worked forty to fifty hours a week and his mother stayed home to care for him. He described his mother as "a helicopter mom" and shared how she would rarely allow him to leave her sight. Alex said he would cry often when his mother would drop him off at kindergarten and elementary school. When his father was around, he would show interest in Alex's intellectual pursuits, but rarely hugged him and would get stern and annoyed when Alex would have a tantrum.

Alex said he felt like he was more open about his emotions in his first couple of romantic relationships, but that he received a lot of negative feedback from his partners who told him he was "too clingy." He identified these experiences as very painful and said he started keeping his feelings to himself more and more.

Alex said that when he met his current partner, things were different. He felt safe with her and she encouraged him to be more open with how he was feeling. Alex said he wanted to be more emotionally expressive with his partner, but whenever she asked how he was feeling, he felt an inner wall go up, leaving him numb and unsure of what he was actually feeling. He reported feeling increasingly distant from his partner and yet deeply longed for a way to feel closer to her.

After spotting how Alex's parts were using outdated strategies, can you identify more of your own? Remember, there's no judgment here. Your inner system of parts was remarkably intuitive in determining what you needed to feel safe and *connected* in your family environment. We encourage you to observe your parts without judgment, understand their motives, and ultimately express appreciation for their hard work in keeping you safe. Don't worry. We'll guide you in learning how to do just that!

Conclusion

This chapter explored the importance of emotional attunement from caregivers in shaping attachment styles. Secure attachment develops when caregivers meet our emotional needs, while insecure attachment—anxious, avoidant, or fearful-avoidant—arises when they do not. These attachment patterns influence our adult relationships.

To maintain connection with caregivers, we develop strategies and behaviors, referred to as "parts" in the IFS model.

In chapter 3, we'll delve into mindfulness to help you understand and work with your internal system of parts. Through exercises, reflections, and teachings, you'll build self-awareness, emotional well-being, and inner harmony.

CHAPTER 3

Going Inside

As we stated in the previous chapter, much of the way we make sense of the world around us and understand our place in it comes from our internal working model, a model that was heavily shaped by early childhood experiences. As a result, our past experiences influence how we respond to current situations. Whether that means we get caught up in trying to predict the future or trying to redo the past, rarely are we actually in the *present moment*. That's not necessarily a bad thing. It's just how our nervous system has evolved to try and keep us safe (more on that in chapter 4!).

However, in this chapter, we're going to look at ways you can safely begin to work with your internal parts and be okay with whatever arises physically, emotionally, and mentally without becoming overwhelmed and shutting down. We invite you to take the time to follow the skills outlined in this chapter one by one. To further assist you in this process, recordings of each guided meditation will be made available online at http://www.newharbinger.com/55909.

Keep in mind that it takes time and practice to learn how to read and interpret the signals from your mind and body, but it is this very practice that can help you truly connect to your parts and provide them with the love and support they didn't receive in childhood.

Blending: Lost in Time

When you view your current experiences through the lens of early childhood memories, it can feel as though you are reliving those past events, even if the present situation is different. If your emotional response feels extreme or out of place in response to the current event, it often originates from a younger part of you. The IFS model calls this *blending* with an internal part. This means you suddenly start experiencing your current situation from the perspective of an internal part that is referencing a similar experience in your life. Which makes some sense: Stick with what worked before. Why reinvent the wheel, right?

The problem here is that the thinking from these parts is "This feels familiar! I know how to take care of this!" as opposed to "That reminds me of something that I survived as a kid. Let me use all of the experiences I've had since then to respond to this completely new and unique situation." Also, the reference points that our parts are relying on are not always clear to us at the moment, which can result in some pretty surprising reactions to seemingly everyday occurrences. For example, your friend might say something to you that reminds you of being bullied in second grade and you yell "Shut up!" In that moment, your reaction is not coming from the adult you who made it through that difficult period of bullying, but from that younger part who thinks that you are suddenly being bullied again.

Your reactions when blended with a part can be dramatic, like exploding in rage or bursting into tears. Or they can be subtle, such as a change in the tone of your voice or shift in body language. Perhaps there's a pattern of behavior you're aware of but haven't had success in changing. For example, you might notice that every time your mother calls, you find yourself getting annoyed before you even answer the phone. You promise yourself you won't let her affect you this time, but once again, you end the call feeling angry at yourself for how you behaved.

If you recognize any of these experiences, you know they can be confusing and disruptive. To make matters worse, when a part blends with you, it often happens without your being aware of it. This can leave you feeling like you got caught up in a trance. When you snap out of it later you might wonder *What just happened? Why did I behave that way?* This is because parts tend to show up with a sense of urgency. From the perspective of your parts, you're still the same age as you were when they first came up with this reaction, so you couldn't possibly know how to take care of yourself. The reasons for this are rooted in your survival instincts, something that we will cover in the next chapter. For now, it's just important to know that when parts blend with you, they take you out of the current moment and limit your ability to respond in the present.

It's important to note that blending is a common experience. It happens to all of us. In fact, most of us move throughout our days with our parts coming in and out of the driver's seat and we are none the wiser! By slowing down and turning inward, we can begin to see how and why our parts blend with us. Once we are in our adult Self, we can reparent our parts, take ownership of our actions, and choose how to respond, rather than feel controlled by our thoughts and behaviors.

Unblending

Just as we can blend with our internal parts, it is also possible to unblend from our parts. *Unblending* is the process of separating from the part's physical, emotional, and mental experiences. When you are blended with a part, your view of the situation narrows down to that part's perspective. However, when you unblend from this part, you can step back and see the situation from a broader, more balanced viewpoint—one that reflects the full context of your life. You are no longer limited to responding as if you are reliving a similar situation from years ago.

Unblending is like directing your own internal movie—zooming out to see the whole scene instead of focusing on one character. This broader perspective helps you recognize all contributing factors, freeing you from past interpretations and allowing fresh, original responses.

Here's an example of unblending by first observing your experience and then grounding yourself in the present moment: After Gabby's first date, her follow-up text went unanswered. Each time she thought about it, her chest tightened, her heart raced, she began sweating, and if she thought about it long enough, she started feeling nauseous. Gabby was blended with an anxious part and was feeling all the sensations of that anxious part.

She decided to pause and take some slow, deep breaths in and out. She realized that she was blended with this part and reassured the part that they were not alone, that she was there with them. Gabby noticed how quickly her body began to relax after doing this. She still did not know why the person had not communicated with her, but when she paid attention to her anxious part, she felt calmer and more confident in her ability to take care of herself, regardless of the outcome.

When we unblend from our parts, the qualities of our true Self naturally emerge, revealing a treasure trove of inner resources. We can then use these resources (*calm, compassion, curiosity*) to heal our parts and begin to respond more effectively to our daily stressors. All of this is possible when we take a pause.

We encourage you to take a pause right now. Can you think of a time when you reacted in a way you didn't understand or regretted? If so, write that down.

_____

_____

_____

_____

Does seeing that reaction as blending with a part change your understanding?

_____

_____

_____

_____

Have you ever experienced the sensation of unblending as described above, even if you were not yet aware of what was happening?

Going Inside

Often the first step to unblending is going inside to be able to track physical sensations, emotions, and thoughts. But what does it mean to "go inside"? And why would we want to?

Going inside simply means shifting your attention from your external environment to focus on your internal experience of bodily sensations, images, thoughts, emotions, or voices that arise within you. Going inside also allows you to tap into your unique inner wisdom—the deep, personal understanding of yourself that only *you* possess. After all, you're the only version of you on the entire planet!

Internal parts hold unresolved emotions, burdens, and past traumas. By practicing the skills of going inside, you learn to regulate your feelings, identify your parts, and learn to work with them. Working with your parts helps you gain *clarity* about why you feel and behave in the ways that you do.

Have you ever had the experience of saying something to someone and immediately hearing a voice in your head exclaim, *Why did you say* that? or *Oh no, what will they think of you now?!* Those are examples of parts communicating with you. If those examples sound familiar in some way, then you're already partially in tune with your inner world.

Mindfulness: Four Tenets

In our experience, one of the most accessible and effective methods for beginning to know our parts is through the practice of mindfulness. Rooted in thousands of years of spiritual practice and tradition, *mindfulness* provides a powerful, secular foundation for doing deep work with your internal system of parts.

As we start working with our internal system, we'll begin to notice that our parts are usually trying to protect us from something. They are either working to prevent potential discomfort or reacting to current discomfort on our behalf. When we are blended with our parts, we become limited to that part's narrow way of handling the situation. Mindfulness provides simple and effective techniques for unblending from these protective parts. It allows us to take in the whole big picture of life and choose for ourselves how we want to respond to any situation, instead of always viewing the world around us as a threat.

But *what is* mindfulness? You may have heard the word mindfulness before, especially if you've taken a yoga or meditation class. The concept of mindfulness has its origins in Hindu and Buddhist traditions dating back thousands of years. Jon Kabat-Zinn (2013, xxvii) has described mindfulness as "paying attention, on purpose, in the present moment, nonjudgmentally." Using Kabat-Zinn's definition of mindfulness, we'll focus on four key principles we find particularly helpful when working with the IFS model: *focused attention, open awareness, observing without judging,* and *kind attention.* These principles come from the Buddhist tradition of Vipassana meditation. *Vipassana* means "to see things as they are." We've highlighted how these practices can help you tap into aspects of Self in italics.

Focus on one tenet or meditation at a time. Take your time with each concept and practice each meditation multiple times before moving to the next. This approach will help you fully internalize each one and integrate it into your daily life. As you become familiar with each, you'll identify which practices are most beneficial for you.

There's no right way to do these exercises—really. If you wonder *Am I doing this right?* or think *I'm getting it wrong!* those may be internal parts speaking. No need to engage—just notice them. Whatever you experience is exactly what needs to happen. Simply doing these exercises lays the groundwork for deeper internal work. Since IFS is experiential, true benefit comes from practicing, not just reading. We've provided a sample meditation tracker here and online at http://www.newharbinger.com/55909 to help you monitor your progress as you move through this chapter.

Meditation Tracker

Day and Time: _____	Day and Time: _____
Duration: _____	Duration: _____
Meditation Type: _____	Meditation Type: _____
Feeling Before: _____	Feeling Before: _____
Feeling After: _____	Feeling After: _____
Notes/Insights: _____	Notes/Insights: _____
_____	_____
_____	_____
Day and Time: _____	Day and Time: _____
Duration: _____	Duration: _____
Meditation Type: _____	Meditation Type: _____
Feeling Before: _____	Feeling Before: _____
Feeling After: _____	Feeling After: _____
Notes/Insights: _____	Notes/Insights: _____
_____	_____
_____	_____

Day and Time: _____

Duration: _____

Meditation Type: _____

Feeling Before: _____

Feeling After: _____

Notes/Insights: _____

_____

_____

Day and Time: _____

Duration: _____

Meditation Type: _____

Feeling Before: _____

Feeling After: _____

Notes/Insights: _____

_____

_____

Day and Time: _____

Duration: _____

Meditation Type: _____

Feeling Before: _____

Feeling After: _____

Notes/Insights: _____

_____

_____

Day and Time: _____

Duration: _____

Meditation Type: _____

Feeling Before: _____

Feeling After: _____

Notes/Insights: _____

_____

_____

Okay, ready? Let's give it a try!

Tenet #1: Focused Attention

Focused attention is the ability to concentrate on one thing at a time, such as your breath. It teaches you to learn to let go of distractions as they arise. This practice helps anchor your mind and brings *clarity* and *calm*.

A helpful technique for practicing focused attention is belly breathing (see below). This practice can help you become aware of how often your mind wanders. Mind wandering is not a bad thing. It is simply a sign that you might not be fully present. If you're not fully present, you may be reacting to the situation from the perspective of a younger version of yourself—a part of you—rather than your adult Self.

Belly Breathing Meditation

Find a quiet place where you can lie down for a few minutes undisturbed. If you like, you can close your eyes to help you focus more inside. If you prefer to leave your eyes open, we recommend finding a place in front of you to look at and then allowing your eyes to go out of focus so as not to get too distracted by the outside world.

Once you're comfortably situated, place both hands on your belly. Direct your attention to the palms of your hands. Feel the movement of your belly as it gently rises with each inhale and as it gently falls with each exhale. See if it's possible to keep your mind focused on the sensation of your belly rising and falling. Each time you notice your mind wandering (and you will, don't worry!), just gently guide your thoughts back to the belly rising and falling. You can think of your thoughts like a small child wandering off and you are just gently guiding them back on track.

Stay with what you are observing for a few more minutes, then when you're ready, gently open your eyes and come to a seated position.

How was that experience?

Did it feel natural?

Was it super hard?

Were you judging yourself?

Do you notice any new sensations?

Has your mood shifted from when you started this exercise?

Take a little time to jot down your experience.

_____

_____

_____

_____

_____

_____

_____

The point of this practice is *not* to keep your thoughts focused on your belly! The purpose of this practice is to learn how to observe with *curiosity*. You're just noticing how often your thoughts wander and maybe beginning to get some idea of where your thoughts might be wandering off to. In addition, it can also be a powerful tool for calming anxiety.

Now, let's transition into the next mindfulness tenet: open awareness.

Tenet #2: Open Awareness

Open awareness teaches you to observe and be present to multiple things at once, such as sensations, thoughts, and emotions, while not getting caught up in or distracted by any one thing. Instead, you can remain *curious* about what you notice and maintain a more zoomed-out perspective on your inner system of parts.

Open Awareness Meditation

Begin by bringing your attention to your breath. Notice the sensation of the air as it enters and leaves your body. Feel the rise and fall of your abdomen with each breath. There is no need to change your breathing; simply observe it as it is.

As you continue to breathe naturally, allow your awareness to expand. Notice the sensations in your body. Feel the weight of your body supported by what you are sitting on. Become aware of the points of contact between your body and the surface you are sitting on. Feel the texture of your clothing against your skin.

Now, expand your awareness to include the sounds around you. Without seeking any particular sound, simply notice what you hear. It might be the hum of the air conditioner, the distant sound of traffic, or the chirping of birds. Allow these sounds to come and go without judgment. Simply observe them as they are.

Next, bring your awareness to your thoughts. Notice any thoughts that arise without getting caught up in them. Notice if you can observe your thoughts as if they were clouds passing through the sky. They come and go, and you remain the observer, *calm* and centered.

Now, allow your awareness to expand even further to include your emotions. Notice any feelings or emotions present within you. Acknowledge them without trying to change them. Simply observe and allow them to be. If you don't notice any, that's okay too.

As you sit in this open awareness, recognize that all these sensations, sounds, thoughts, and emotions are part of your present-moment experience. There is no need to cling to any of them or push them away. They are all part of the rich tapestry of this moment.

Take a few more deep breaths, feeling a sense of *connection* to the space around you. Know that you can return to this state of open awareness at any time, simply by tuning in to your breath and observing your experience with gentle *curiosity* and acceptance.

When you feel ready, gently bring your awareness back to your body and the space you are in. Wiggle your fingers and toes, and when you're ready, slowly open your eyes.

How was that for you?

Were there any thoughts that tried to distract you?

What about strong sensations?

Or strong feelings?

These may be coming from parts. As you learn to simply observe, you create a little distance, which is a form of unblending.

Tenet #3: Observing Without Judging

Have you ever noticed how quickly your mind can jump into judging others or yourself? For example, you might hear yourself say *Why is she wearing that outfit? It's so ugly!* or *I'll never succeed if I don't toughen up.* If so, don't beat yourself up. We all have parts that try to protect us by making value judgments—about either others' thoughts and behaviors or our own.

However, harsh self-criticism or criticism of others often leads to a cycle of stress and anxiety. Judging others can also create a false sense of superiority, which may cause you to distance yourself from others and feel more isolated. Judgment, whether toward yourself or others, fosters negativity, limits joy, and hinders personal and relational growth by creating barriers to understanding and acceptance.

What are the first three things that come to mind when you think about judging yourself?

_____

_____

_____

What are the first three things that come to mind when you think about judging others?

_____

_____

_____

What does it feel like to recognize your judgments of others? Do you notice thoughts like *It's not fair to judge others* or feelings of shame or self-criticism?

_____

_____

_____

_____

Can you imagine what it would be like to be free from your self-judgment?

_____

_____

_____

See if you can rewrite the three things you wrote about judging yourself in a more *compassionate* and nonjudgmental way, such as "That was how I acted that one time, not who I am all the time" or "That was a tough moment for me and I did what I could to get through it."

_____

_____

_____

_____

_____

Now, see if you can do the same thing with the three things you wrote about judging others, such as "Everyone has different tastes in clothing, music, food, and so on, and that's okay" or "I wonder what was going on for them that made them act that way?"

_____

_____

_____

_____

_____

MINDFUL EXERCISE: Observing Without Judging

Think of a time when you were judging yourself or someone else. Bring to mind as much detail as possible. Where were you? What was happening? What were you wearing? Who was there? See if you can remember what you were saying about yourself or that other person that felt judgmental. How did it feel in your body as you were being judgmental? Did you feel better, worse, or neutral afterward? Write down everything that you remember below.

_____

_____

_____

_____

_____

Now, imagine revisiting that moment with acceptance instead. How would it feel to accept yourself or that person just as they are? If you find that difficult, what do you notice instead? What thoughts, feelings, or sensations show up when you try to accept versus judge? What are you afraid would happen if you didn't judge that person? Take a moment to write down what you notice about practicing acceptance.

_____

_____

_____

_____

_____

_____

How was that exercise in trying to cultivate a nonjudgmental attitude? It's okay if it was challenging. Practicing something new is challenging for everyone! Learning how to be nonjudgmental is a living, ongoing practice we can do every single day. And it's worth the effort!

Practicing nonjudgment encourages a soft, open acceptance of things as they truly are, without feeling the need to change them. When you begin to notice your reactions as opposed to labeling them as "good" or "bad," you may find that the habit of judging starts to ease on its own. Accepting reality as it is—instead of how you wish it were—helps you let go of judgments that arise from resistance or denial. This kind of open acceptance makes space for you to connect with all parts of yourself from a place of *curiosity* without the need to change them.

When you learn to offer yourself *compassion* and self-acceptance, including all parts of who you are, this allows you to extend the same to others. This shift not only improves your state of mind but also transforms how you *connect* with others. You begin to interact with greater kindness, especially with those you care about most—and they can sense it. Though simple, this practice can deepen your relationships by fostering greater trust and intimacy. Building deeper *connections* is a key part of creating a more fulfilling life in a world often marked by loneliness.

Tenet #4: Kind Attention

Kind attention is the practice of maintaining a positive, *compassionate*, and loving state of mind. This attitude can be directed both toward others and toward yourself, fostering a sense of warmth and *connection* in all aspects of your life. We find meditations that encourage "unconditional positive regard," a term coined by the humanistic psychotherapist Carl Rogers (1961), to be most effective at helping us *connect* with our inner Self and with others.

Compassionate Being Meditation

Think of someone or something, whether real or imagined, that accepts you completely. It could be a person, a pet, a fictional character, a spiritual being, whatever brings to mind the sense that this person, thing, or being can accept you exactly as you are.

Once you have your being in mind, imagine that they are there with you right now. Imagine they are looking at you with warmth, love, and familiarity. Feel their presence there with you and notice how that impacts your mood, your thoughts, and how you feel in your body. Stay here as long as you like.

Now, shift your imagination to a recent event that was embarrassing, scary, stressful, or uncomfortable in some way. Nothing too upsetting, but just enough to notice some discomfort. Once you've identified the event, try to remember as much detail as possible. Imagine you are back in the actual event as if it were happening *right now*. Notice how you feel in comparison to how you felt in the presence of your compassionate being. Was there a sudden shift? Or was it gradual? Did any new thoughts arise as you shifted your imagination to the uncomfortable event? Did you notice any emotions or physical sensations in your body when remembering the uncomfortable event? These thoughts, feelings, or sensations may be parts. Whatever is here, see if you can simply observe it as opposed to feeling caught up in it.

Now, as you stay with that uncomfortable event, imagine your compassionate being reappearing while you are experiencing it. They do not change any of the details, but simply look at you with the same warmth and acceptance as before. You are aware of their presence even as you go through this uncomfortable experience. Notice if this changes how you experience this memory. Are your thoughts the same as before or different? Does your view of your reaction to the situation change at all? Do you feel different in your body as you imagine your compassionate being witnessing you go through this uncomfortable experience? Again, there's no need for any specific response. Simply observe what happened. When you are ready, gently return your attention to your surroundings in the present. Take some time to write down what came up for you during this meditation.

_____

_____

_____

_____

_____

_____

In many ways, this compassionate being resembles what the IFS model refers to as the Self. The only difference is that instead of another person embodying the characteristics of Self (*calm, curiosity, compassion, creativity, clarity, courage, confidence,* and *connectedness*), *you* contain all of these attributes inside of you. This is just one example of a way you might begin to reparent yourself with the qualities of Self. Let's move on to another meditation that can foster aspects of Self: Originally referred to as *metta* in the Pali language, this Buddhist meditation was introduced by Sharon Salzberg in 1995 as the "loving-kindness meditation."

Loving-Kindness Meditation

Our suggestion during this meditation is to track the parts of yourself that appear with each prompt. Notice which parts show up when you offer *compassion* to yourself, to a loved one, to a stranger, and so on. This practice helps you understand how your different parts respond to *compassion,* deepening your self-awareness and empathy.

Gently close your eyes or allow your eyes to go slightly out of focus. Take a few deep breaths. Inhale deeply through your nose and exhale slowly through your mouth. Allow your breathing to return to its natural rhythm. Feel the rise and fall of your chest and abdomen with each breath.

Begin by directing loving-kindness toward yourself. Either out loud or silently to yourself, repeat the following phrases three times each:

- May I be happy.

- May I be healthy.

- May I be safe.

- May I live with ease.

As you say these phrases, try to generate a warm and loving feeling toward yourself. Visualize yourself surrounded by a warm, glowing light.

Next, bring to mind someone you care about deeply. Visualize this person clearly in your mind and repeat the phrases to them:

- May you be happy.

- May you be healthy.

- May you be safe.

- May you live with ease.

Imagine this person surrounded by a warm, glowing light, filled with your loving kindness.

Think of someone you see regularly but don't have strong feelings for, like a coworker or a neighbor. Visualize them and repeat the same phrases: "May he/she/they be happy," and so on.

Bring to mind someone with whom you have a challenging relationship. This can be someone who has upset you or wronged you in some way. If you like, you can focus on a part of yourself that you may not like. This might be difficult, but try to send them loving-kindness as well. Repeat the same phrases for them.

Finally, extend your loving-kindness to all beings everywhere. Visualize the entire world and all living beings within it. Repeat the same phrases: "May all beings everywhere be happy," and so on.

Take a few deep breaths. Slowly bring your awareness back to the present moment. Notice details of the space around you that feel familiar in order to ground you back in the present. Take a moment to notice how you feel after this practice.

How was that for you? Were there any moments that stood out to you? As you moved through the practice, first focusing on yourself and then others, did you notice any thoughts, emotions, physical sensations, or impulses? Was there a voice inside telling you that this was silly or a waste of time? Did you have an itch that you had to scratch? Or a need to keep shifting your body to get more comfortable? Or nothing at all?

As you review your experience, take a moment to write down what you noticed about each area of focus. Any tidbit of information could be useful as a hint about a part that might have showed up while you were engaged in this activity, so feel free to jot down everything, even if it doesn't totally make sense.

Yourself: _____

_____

_____

_____

_____

Person you care about: _____

_____

_____

_____

_____

Neutral person: _____

_____

_____

_____

_____

Challenging person: _____

_____

_____

_____

_____

All beings everywhere: _____

_____

_____

_____

_____

Conclusion

At this point, we hope you're beginning to feel more comfortable with the concept of internal parts and starting to notice how they show up in your daily life. You now have a variety of mindfulness tools to choose from. As you try each one multiple times, you may start to identify your favorites. By practicing these mindfulness techniques, you'll build a set of tools and resources to guide and support you as you continue this inner work. You can access a chart with a link to all of these meditations online at http://www.newharbinger.com/55909.

In chapter 4, we'll transition from the land of the mind into the realm of the body! We will build on the resources you've already learned to help teach you how to fully connect with your body and pay attention to messages and signals from your body that can guide you toward a greater understanding of your internal system. Developing these skills is essential for learning how to engage with your internal parts. We're excited to guide you through these steps and will be right here to support you along the way.

CHAPTER 4

Connecting
to the Body

As we stated in the previous chapter, mindfulness helps us to be where our bodies are in the present moment as opposed to where our minds *think* we are. At this point, you might be thinking, *What is so important about connecting to our bodies?* Great question!

Besides showing up in our thoughts, our internal parts can also communicate to us through our nervous system as impulses, emotions, and physical sensations. It is extremely important to pay attention to these felt signals from our body and not just ignore them or write them off as irrelevant. These aren't simply sensations. All of these internal and bodily sensations are opportunities to look inward and understand ourselves better.

We will be teaching you a series of body-based exercises to help you understand how you feel emotions in your body and provide you with tools to help regulate your nervous system. These skills will support you as you begin to identify and work with your internal parts in the following chapters.

Body-Mind Connection

Many of us are caught up in our thoughts, often prioritizing the mind while neglecting the body. Maybe you value rational thought and logic, and think "illogical" or "irrational" emotions get in the way of happiness? Or maybe you're stuck in operation mode to get through every day? As a result, you live in your head, disconnected from your body unless you're battling an illness. This focus on thought, while not altogether negative, can result in a disregard for all the important ways that your body influences how you view and react to the world around you.

Just as you cannot remove your internal parts, you cannot separate yourself from your body. No amount of rational thinking or logical reasoning can change the fact that you exist and move through the world in a physical body. Jon Kabat-Zinn stated this beautifully in the title of his second book, *Wherever You Go, There You Are* (1994).

Susan McConnell (2020), a senior trainer at the IFS Institute, made a significant contribution to the IFS model by integrating body-based practices referred to as "somatics" (the word "somatics" from the Greek word "soma," meaning "body"). This somatic integration strengthens the model's effectiveness by helping us connect with our inner parts and revisit childhood wounds, allowing for deeper healing.

Take a moment right now to pause and see what you notice in your body. Pay attention to the physical sensations, such as temperature, pressure, and tension. Can you pinpoint the location of these sensations? Are they in one place, all over, or is it unclear? Any response is fine. This is simply a first step in building awareness of the physical sensations your body experiences constantly—many of which go unnoticed. Take a moment to write what you noticed below.

_____

_____

_____

_____

_____

If you find yourself asking _Is this whole body-mind thing really that important?_ we have a little exercise we'd like you to try:

Imagine right now there's an adorable puppy snuggled up next to you. Take a moment and notice how you feel. Are the sensations pleasant, unpleasant, or neutral? Again, how do you feel in your body? What thoughts do you notice coming up? Stay with whatever is coming up for you for a few more moments.

Now, imagine that you suddenly notice a cockroach scurrying up your leg. How do you feel? Are the sensations similar to your reaction to the puppy or are they different? Pleasant, unpleasant, or neutral? We're gonna go out on a limb here and guess that you felt different in your body imagining a puppy versus a cockroach!

Apologies if that exercise stirred up any strong reactions, but we wanted to highlight the impact the imagination (i.e., the mind) has on your body and vice versa. For example, we both felt a warm, calm feeling throughout our bodies when imagining the puppy. That feeling was quickly shattered the second we imagined a cockroach running up our legs. In our bodies, we noticed our heart rate rapidly increased, and we felt a desire to jump up or quickly move our legs even though there was no cockroach there. Happy or painful memories can have this same impact.

Engaging the body through somatic exercises can bring up some surprisingly strong physical and emotional reactions. We encourage you to keep this in mind when following our prompts going forward. If something starts to feel too uncomfortable, intense, or overwhelming, feel free to take a break or skip it for now.

Now that we have opened the door a bit to understanding the body-mind connection, here's an example from Kyle's life to illustrate what we're talking about.

For years, I (Kyle) had a painful pinched nerve in my right shoulder. The pain would shoot down my entire right arm all the way to my pointer finger. Over time, the intensity of the pain grew and became so intense that I stopped using my right arm altogether in the hope that resting it might help the pain subside.

One night, my pinched nerve was so inflamed that I began to feel hopeless and scared that I had caused some kind of irrevocable damage. I was at the end of my rope and desperate for any kind of relief. Luckily, having worked with pain-related parts before, I decided to try and see if there was a part there!

I lay in bed and closed my eyes. Immediately, I was thrust back into a memory from childhood. My father was looking at me very angrily about something and was pinching my shoulder, which is how he tended to show his displeaure. He is left-handed, so he would have been pinching my right shoulder. The intensity of this memory was startling, but I was able to stay with it and help this part share what it was still holding: the belief that I was bad.

Suddenly, a flood of understanding came over me. All those times I felt that pinched nerve getting unbearable were related to moments in my work when I felt like I was not doing a good job. This pinched nerve had a history attached to it!

Now, when I feel that same discomfort starting to show up, it serves as a reminder to slow down and check in with that part. I still get some shoulder discomfort from time to time, but since making that discovery, I have not had another incident of crippling pain and I have even started to appreciate the reminder that part gives me to be less hard on myself.

This story is meant to illustrate how our parts can communicate to us through physical sensations. We're not expecting you to be able to have this level of awareness right off the bat. Instead, we hope you'll feel more motivated to notice the subtle signals from your body and recognize how paying attention to discomfort can actually help you.

Have you ever experienced a physical discomfort or ailment that seemed to arise in specific situations? For example, have you noticed your stomach tightening or a fluttering sensation, like butterflies, when you're feeling anxious—such as before giving a presentation at work or stepping up to bat in a baseball game? Or perhaps you get a headache when anticipating a visit from your in-laws.

We invite you to start paying closer attention to the sensations in your body and the situations in which they arise. These feelings may be connected to a past experience or stem from a part of you that is trying to communicate something. To explore what these sensations might mean on a deeper level, it's essential to first become aware of the physical sensations you notice in your body. Let's start by helping you to notice what's happening in your body *right now!*

Body Scan Meditation

The body scan meditation is a powerful tool for strengthening your physical and mental well-being by fostering a deep connection between body and mind. As you focus on each part of your body, you are practicing a form of mindfulness. Remember, as you engage in paying attention to your thoughts, feelings, and bodily sensations, you are doing so without judgment.

When you begin working with a part, you start by noticing where you find the part *in*, *on*, or *around* your body. As you tune in to your body, you may notice how *emotions* manifest as physical sensations: a tightness in the chest or clenching of the jaw. Recognizing this connection helps you determine if the emotion is coming from a part stuck in the past. As you learn to quickly scan your body, you'll locate your parts more readily with practice.

Let's begin: The key here is to move your awareness slowly and mindfully, staying present with each part of your body as you scan from head to toe.

Find a quiet space where you won't be disturbed. You can sit or lie down, whichever feels more comfortable for you. Close your eyes if you like.

Take a few deep breaths, inhaling through your nose and exhaling through your mouth. Feel the air filling your lungs and notice the rise and fall of your chest and abdomen with each breath. Allow your breath to settle into a natural rhythm.

Start by noticing the points of contact between your body and the surface you're resting on. Feel the weight of your body being supported. Shift your attention to your toes. Feel each toe individually, and notice any sensations—warmth, tingling, or even numbness.

Slowly move your awareness up through your feet, noticing the soles, arches, and heels. Continue up through your ankles, calves, and shins. What sensations do you notice?

Move your awareness up to your knees and thighs. Notice the muscles and any areas of tightness or ease. Next, bring your focus to your hips and pelvis. Notice how they feel, the points of contact with the surface beneath you, and any sensations that arise.

Continue as you shift your attention to your lower back and abdomen, feeling the gentle rise and fall of your belly with each breath. Move your awareness up to your upper back and chest. Notice any areas of tension or stress. Shift your focus on your shoulders. What do you notice here? Are there any thoughts or emotions that seem located here? What about in your upper arms, elbows, forearms, wrists, hands, and fingers?

Bring your attention to your neck and throat. Notice the natural curve of your neck, and the feeling of your breath moving through your throat. Is it tight or soft? Gently move up to your face.

Notice your jaw, cheeks, nose, eyes, and forehead. What are you aware of here? Finally, move your awareness to the top of your head, noticing any sensations there.

Now, take a moment to sense your entire body as a whole, from the tips of your toes to the top of your head.

When you're ready, gently wiggle your fingers and toes, bringing a little movement back into your body. Slowly open your eyes and take a moment to notice how you feel before moving on with your day.

How was that for you? Did you notice anything surprising? Familiar? Confusing? Upsetting? Were there places of tension? Did your mind wander when scanning over certain areas of your body? Did certain areas of your body bring up negative feelings? Or positive feelings? Did you have any memories that showed up? Perhaps a desire to move your body in some way? Whatever you noticed, take some time right now to jot it down here.

_____

_____

_____

_____

_____

_____

_____

_____

_____

The Nervous System

Now that we've done a body scan, let's learn about another important aspect of the body-mind connection, the role of the nervous system. We'll start by introducing clinical researcher Stephen Porges's research on the mammalian nervous system.

The Vagus Nerve and Neuroception

Conventional science sees the autonomic nervous system (ANS) as having two main branches: the sympathetic and parasympathetic. The sympathetic nervous system controls the body's *fight or flight response*. The parasympathetic nervous system helps control your body's response during rest, what is known as *rest and digest functions*. Stephen Porges suggests a third branch of the nervous system that he labels the "ventral vagal complex" (VVC), which is also part of the parasympathetic nervous system (2011). According to Dr. Porges, the VVC is part of the vagus nerve, which lets mammals co-regulate, bond, and form complex social relationships (2003). It coordinates heart rate with facial and head muscles to enable *social engagement,* through eye gaze, vocalization, head turning, and facial expression, all of which are critical for feeling safe and *connected* with others. He theorizes that this branch of the nervous system is the latest evolutionary update and is unique to mammals. When we can orient and *connect* with other mammals in a safe and calming way, we use this branch of the nervous system. For example, if you were at a park and saw a threatening person approaching your baby, you might lock eyes with another parent and quickly ask for help to protect your child. By doing so, you engage the social connection branch.

Our bodies have nervous systems that have evolved over millions of years to do some pretty incredible things. Your nervous system has guided your development from the time you were a tiny baby to the point where you can now read and understand the words on this page. That alone is incredible!

Another incredible fact is how communication flows between the brain and the body. The vagus nerve, which is actually a bundle of nerves, starts in the brainstem and travels down through the neck and chest into the abdomen, branching out to connect with major organs like the heart, lungs, and digestive tract (Standring 2015). It plays a central role in helping our brains interpret and respond to everything happening inside and outside our bodies. Remarkably, about 80 percent of the information from the nervous system travels from the body to the brain, while only 20 percent of the signals travel from the brain to the body (Howland 2014). This means that, much of the time, we react to life through instinctive, body-based responses rather than through deliberate, rational thinking.

To help you understand how you might notice this in your body, think about a time when you were crossing the street and suddenly a car came speeding toward you. How did you react? Did you stop and think, *Hmm, that's a car. What should I do? I guess I'll jump out of the way...* Or did you simply jump out of the way? Our guess is the latter. Your body sensed danger and knew instinctively how to save you in that moment.

Our body's automatic response is guided by a system that continuously monitors our surroundings, preparing us to react instinctively to potential threats or signs of safety. Without our being consciously aware of it, our ANS is rapidly categorizing everything into one of three groups: safe, dangerous, or life-threatening. This process, known as *neuroception*, is entirely unconscious and is happening all the time (Porges 2004).

The example of crossing the street is a great example of neuroception at work. Without your even thinking about it, your nervous system registered that you were in danger and instinctually mobilized you to get out of danger. Neuroception happens every second of every day and can influence how you experience the world and the people around you. This constant, unconscious process plays a crucial role in shaping our attachment experiences by assessing whether our caregiver felt safe or unsafe.

The Nervous System and Attachment

If your caregiver was unable or unwilling to provide attunement, your brain and nervous system instinctively perceived this as danger—and for good reason. As a mammal, your survival depended on staying connected to your caregiver. Without that connection, your nervous system interpreted the lack of attunement as a threat to your very survival.

When the family environment feels unsafe, we lose the opportunity to learn self-soothing and regulation. As a response we often remain in fight, flight, or freeze states. Anxiously attached children may exhibit fight (pursuit) responses, avoidant styles tend toward flight, and disorganized styles may freeze, caught between the fight and flight response simultaneously. From the start, our nervous system tracks safety and danger, shaping these survival responses. Let's do an exercise to help you start identifying your nervous system reactions.

EXERCISE: Protect and Connect

Remember a time when you took an immediate dislike to someone and you couldn't explain why. Maybe they seemed rude or you felt creeped out by their presence. Perhaps you noticed a frown or a scowl on their face. Or you reacted to their tone that seemed harsh or judgmental. Take a moment to write down the example that comes to mind.

_____

_____

_____

_____

As you remember that experience, what do you notice in your body?

_____

_____

_____

Now, take a moment to think about a time when you felt an instant _connection_ with someone. Maybe it was their warm smile that made you feel at ease, the tone of their voice that felt comforting, or the genuine interest they showed in what you were saying. Reflect on that experience and write about it below.

_____

_____

_____

_____

Focusing exclusively on the physical sensations you experienced in your body, how did the two experiences differ? What signals did your body give you to communicate a need for protection? What signals did your body give you to communicate a willingness for *connection*?

_____

_____

_____

_____

This exercise demonstrates how we can shift from a state of protection to *connection*. The moment you stop feeling safe, your nervous system instantly switches from being open to *connection* to being on high alert. It begins to view everything and everyone as a potential threat. Once this happens, we start to feel a sense of urgency, and it becomes much harder to stay *calm* and respond thoughtfully.

This heightened sense of urgency is deeply tied to early experiences of perceived danger, which become embedded in our brain, nervous system, and body as unconscious memories. As babies and toddlers, our brain was still developing the ability to store conscious memories, so these early impressions remain below our awareness when we are adults. Instead of being stored as images and words we can consciously remember and explain later—known as *explicit* memory (e.g., "that happened because of this")—experiences that the nervous system sees as critical for survival are stored as *implicit* memories, which are unconscious and felt in the body rather than recalled with words. As opposed to the *details* of the experience being stored in the brain, they are stored as physical sensations and reactions that occurred *at the time of the original threat*. In other words, if something reminds us of a painful experience in the past, we may feel it in our body as opposed to being reminded of a specific event.

Let's say you have an argument with your partner. Without warning, your body shuts down. Your mind goes blank and you can't speak. Chances are, you are getting triggered by an implicit memory. Your brain, nervous system, and body are referencing a childhood memory without your realizing it. Without your conscious awareness, your brain is likely drawing on a *felt* experience from early childhood. This implicit memory is activating and triggering a threat response in your nervous system.

As infants and children, we depended on our caregivers to help us regulate our emotions because we couldn't do it on our own. When our caregivers couldn't provide this support, we found ways to soothe ourselves, doing whatever we could to cope. Maybe we turned to sweet or salty foods to help us feel better in the moment. Or maybe we found TV to be an effective distraction from lack of attunement. Perhaps we ran around the house in an effort to burn off excess energy. Whatever we did, the self-soothing strategies we developed as children may no longer serve us—or may not be the only ways we can regulate ourselves now. The good news is that, as adults, we can learn to provide ourselves with the attunement, *connection*, and support we may not have received when we needed them most.

Take a moment to pause and consider this: What are some ways you self-soothe?

_____

_____

_____

_____

_____

_____

_____

These self-soothing strategies often developed in response to painful or traumatic childhood experiences. When the emotional pain felt too overwhelming to manage alone, parts may have learned to suppress their feelings and emotions. The problem is, emotion is a type of energy and ignoring or suppressing that energy doesn't make it go away. Instead, it can get trapped in our body and nervous system.

The Emotional Connection

Where do emotions fit into the body-mind connection? We feel emotions in the body, but they can be hard to identify—often appearing as tension, warmth, or a surge of energy, especially with fear or anger. Interestingly, there is an overlap between emotional and physical pain in certain areas of the brain (Fogel 2012). This overlap helps explain why emotional pain, such as social rejection or grief, can feel physically distressing.

You may have heard another common expression these days: "I have an *emotional hangover!*" Neuroscience demonstrates that emotional states can linger for an extended period of time after an emotional event. Think of the pain that comes with an intense argument, break-up, a heart-ache. You don't shake that in a few hours! It's visceral. You *feel* it in your body and it's tiring and draining the next day and even for days and weeks afterward.

The IFS model calls these intense emotional states being *flooded*. In other words, a part is flooding our body with emotion to the point of overwhelm. What do we do with such strong sensations and feelings? After all, we humans don't want to feel pain. We instinctively retract and withdraw from discomfort, whether it's physical or emotional.

When we experience emotions in a grounded, present way, we feel balanced. But many of us haven't felt safe enough to process emotions healthily. In unsafe childhood environments, we may have retreated into our mind or trapped emotions in our body. For instance, when I (Martina) was a child, I regularly suppressed speaking my mind, which led to chronic tightness in my throat, jaw, and neck. Later, as my parts learned it was safe to express what I was feeling, this chronic tightness resolved.

I (Martina) was a sensitive child. I can remember feeling frequently hurt and rejected by my peers. I unconsciously learned to slump my shoulders to hide my heart. I also had chronic belly aches from feeling so much anger and clenched my belly to hold it in.

Can you relate to any of the examples above? It's very common to carry persistent tension or tightness in certain areas of your body. This tension is often linked to an emotional response from different parts of you. In many cases, it's related to a fight, flight, or freeze reaction stored in the body. When emotions are suppressed or ignored rather than processed, they don't just disap-pear. Emotional responses can become "trapped" in the body when we experience overwhelming or unresolved emotions, especially during stress or trauma. Strong emotions trigger physiological responses like increased heart rate and muscle tension. If these emotions aren't fully processed, the body retains this tension. Suppressing emotions like anger (fight) or fear (flight) can leave the physiological charge of those emotions trapped in the body.

Can you remember a time in childhood this happened to you? If so, write it down:

_____

_____

_____

_____

_____

What did it feel like to have to keep the emotion inside?

_____

_____

_____

_____

Was there a time you wanted to run away from something, but you couldn't?

_____

_____

_____

_____

_____

Do you remember a time in childhood when you held in your emotions rather than expressed them? If so, when you think of that memory, do you notice any tension in your body? Where?

_____

_____

_____

_____

Are there some areas where you hold constant tension or tightness? These areas can be trailheads in discovering parts that got stuck somatically.

_____

_____

_____

_____

For a fun exercise on where you locate emotions in your body go to the bonus content at http://www.newharbinger.com/55909.

As clinicians, we've observed that when a part becomes stuck in a client's mind, they often disconnect—numbing out or spacing out. When a part is stuck in the body, the emotional response tends to intensify. For instance, hurt may become despair, sadness may deepen into depression, happiness may escalate into mania, anger may flare into rage, and rejection may feel like abandonment. Instead of judging these reactions, we can view them as natural responses shaped by challenging early experiences.

To do parts work successfully, we need to be willing to see and witness the painful wounds and stuck emotions our younger parts carry. When we offer this in support, the part is able to process and resolve them. It will become important to increase our comfort level—or "window of tolerance"—in order to tolerate our emotions and accompanying physical discomfort. This is known as *emotional regulation*, which involves learning how to experience and respond to our emotions in a way that helps process and resolve them.

If emotions can disrupt our internal system, you might wonder why we have them at all. Let's explore that question next.

Why Nature Gave Us Emotions

We can't tell you how many clients tell us that emotions or feelings are stupid, useless, and that they just get in the way. Why such a negative view? Well, perhaps our families didn't model healthy emotional processing—we were punished for showing emotion or emotions were seen as irrational or "too much."

Why, then, did Mother Nature give us emotions? Just to play a trick on us? It sure seems that way sometimes!

As therapists, we believe emotions are resources. Emotions provide valuable information, guide decision-making, motivate action, and reveal our thoughts, needs, and desires. For example, longing for love drives many to seek a partner, while unhappiness at work signals a need for change. Guilt prompts us to make amends, and grief helps heal a broken heart after loss. Anger alerts us when boundaries are crossed and motivates self-protection.

As you can see, emotions help us navigate life and strengthen connections. Feelings and emotions are not the problem. The problem is when they are expressed in unhelpful ways. For example, anger is perfectly natural, but if you saw your caretaker express anger in a punitive or rageful way, it felt unsafe. If you learn how to process your emotions through your body and sensations in a helpful manner, you will help these young wounded parts heal. And you will find yourself living a more vibrant, fulfilling life. We get that you may find even the thought of experiencing your emotions to be scary and daunting. We're here to help.

Creating Safety to Process Emotion

Think of standing on a beach where the water serenely laps onto the sand, and imagine in the distance, a big wave is forming. It's large and looks a bit menacing. Yet, we know that as the wave rolls closer and closer to the shore, it will become smaller and smaller.

Look at the diagram and imagine a wave of emotion arising. On a scale of 0 to 10, your emotions rise until they peak at 10 and then begin to slowly subside. Zero might be calm, peaceful, and 5 might be when your emotion starts to become uncomfortable, triggering some agitation or a desire to distract, and 10 might be total panic, rage, or spacing out.

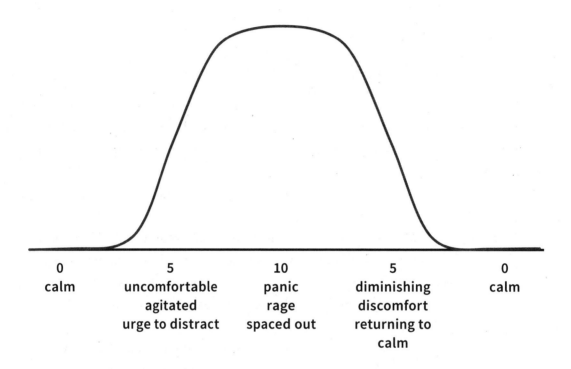

0	5	10	5	0
calm	uncomfortable agitated urge to distract	panic rage spaced out	diminishing discomfort returning to calm	calm

EXERCISE: Riding the Emotional Wave

Think of something that has recently upset you. Bring the memory to mind, allowing yourself to fully feel the emotions connected to it. Write down the memory and emotions.

_____

_____

_____

_____

How high would you rate it on the wave scale? _____

Shift your focus to your body. Can you feel any physical sensations connected to this emotion? It might be tightness in your chest, a lump in your throat, tension in your shoulders, or something else. Take note of where it is and write it down.

_____

_____

_____

_____

Allow yourself to focus on that sensation. Don't try to fight or change it—just let it be. Imagine the sensation growing, intensifying like a wave building in the ocean.

Ride the wave. Visualize yourself as a surfer on a board. As the wave of sensation builds, stay with it. Breathe deeply and evenly as you ride through the discomfort. It may feel strong or overwhelming, but remind yourself that all waves eventually pass.

Notice as the sensation reaches its peak. Stay present. After the peak, the wave will start to descend. Let it carry you down gently. Breathe. Observe the feeling as it softens and calms.

When the wave subsides, take a moment to notice the stillness that follows. Feel the calm in your body and mind. Breathe deeply—you stayed with the emotion, and it has now passed!

How did it feel to ride the wave? Did you notice anything new about the connection between your emotions and your body?

Repeat this exercise whenever you're overwhelmed by strong emotions to practice emotional mindfulness and regulation.

When our emotions are not fully processed, different parts of us tend to hold onto them. For example, a part of you might carry painful memories of feeling embarrassed as a child. If, at that time, a caregiver wasn't available to help you process those emotions or attune to your needs, that part may continue to carry the burden of shame—both emotionally and physically.

In order to reparent the younger internal parts of us, we must first learn how to regulate ourselves in the present. After all, as infants and children, we were unable to regulate our own emotions. We looked to our caregivers for guidance and support on how to do that. If your caregivers were unable to consistently provide a sense of safety and connection, it's important to know that you can now step into that role for yourself. By practicing these self-regulation skills and connecting with aspects of Self (*calm*, *curious*, *compassionate*), *you* can become the ideal, supportive parent you needed. In other words, you can learn to create secure internal attachment and regulate your nervous system in a healthy way.

Conclusion

We hope this introduction to the body-mind connection inspires you to continue exploring this powerful relationship. While your mind may wander, your body remains a steady anchor in the present moment. By gently tuning in to your body, you can deepen self-awareness and build emotional resilience. Many of our feelings stem from parts of us still holding onto the past, reacting to old wounds in the present. By noticing the sensations and emotions within your body, you can begin to connect with these parts and support their healing.

In the next chapter, we'll help you put what you've learned into practice as we begin working with your parts, starting with managers.

CHAPTER 5

Connecting to Your Managers

Congratulations, you've reached the halfway point! So far, you've learned about the IFS model and its structure, explored attachment styles, and learned how childhood experiences influence later behaviors and feelings. You've also learned how to utilize mindfulness and somatic practices to go inside and explore your internal system by paying attention to your thoughts, emotions, and physical sensations.

Take a moment and check in with your internal system. How are you doing right now as you prepare to begin this chapter? Are you feeling more comfortable going inside and exploring your internal world? Or are you still feeling a bit unsure or confused? Maybe a bit of both? Or something else? Take a moment to write down how you're feeling at this juncture.

_____

_____

_____

_____

_____

_____

_____

_____

Wherever you are right now is exactly where you need to be. No one else in history has lived the same life or had the same experiences as you. This makes you uniquely equipped to understand who you are and what you need *in this moment*. No one knows that better than you.

Remember: No single event or experience defines who you are or determines how you should respond to every situation. As you begin working with your internal parts, we encourage you to keep this in mind and trust your unique wisdom.

Let's explore your internal system of protective parts. The parts that tend to appear most often as you navigate daily life are known as the *manager parts*.

Manager Parts

Growing up, we rely on our caregivers to meet not only our physical needs but our emotional ones as well. When a caregiver lacks sufficient access to their own Self-energy, we struggle in childhood to have our emotional needs met in a consistent, nurturing way. Remember: The aspects of Self-energy are characterized by qualities like *compassion*, *calmness*, *clarity*, and *connectedness*, which are essential for our healthy emotional development. If our caregiver is unable to access these qualities, often because of their own unresolved childhood trauma, pain, or difficulties, we struggle to access our own Self-energy.

When we grow up without a Self-led caregiver, we're forced to find ways to fill the emotional gaps ourselves. To ensure our caregiver continues meeting our basic needs—like food, clothing, and shelter—we find ways to stay emotionally connected to them, even if that means suppressing our own needs. But without being seen and emotionally validated, we're often left with insecure attachment, difficulty regulating emotions, and intense feelings of hurt, shame, rejection, or isolation.

How can we possibly cope in such an environment? It's too scary. We feel too vulnerable.

One way we cope is by forming internal protectors. Our first line of defense is what IFS calls manager parts. They protect the most vulnerable parts of us (more on this in chapter 7). These protector parts give up their natural ability to play and simply be children. Instead, they are driven into roles they often dislike in order to keep us safe. Think of a people-pleaser part stepping in so that your caregiver doesn't get so mad they kick you out of the house. The people pleaser can't relax. They have to stay in that role to keep you safe.

Manager parts are called "managers" because they help us *manage* situations. Managers are *proactive* protectors. Their goal is to maintain order. They work hard to prevent us from being hurt or overwhelmed by keeping vulnerable parts from being triggered. These parts of us are constantly on alert, working ahead of time to protect us by spotting and avoiding possible dangers. Because they're so active, they often feel like the most familiar and consistent parts of our personalities. They are also helpful resources. Managers are responsible for helping us function—planning ahead, keeping commitments, appearing "okay"—even when there's pain under the surface. Where would we be if we didn't have a time manager to get us to work on time or a decision-maker manager to help us prioritize daily tasks? The trouble comes in when they take on *extreme* roles, such as an "inner critic" or "worrywart."

Getting to Know a Manager Part

When working with clients and their managers, we often hear things like "That's not a part—that's just me" or "I'm always anxious." These reactions make sense in a way—rather than seeing our behaviors as parts of us that help us navigate life, many of us instead assume they define who we are. We encourage clients to get *curious* about this assumption. Even if an experience seems constant, we ask: "Is this really true all the time?" If the answer is no, there may be space to step back and view that behavior as a part, not the whole self. By asking *How do I feel when I'm not like that?* clients can discover a trailhead—a valuable starting point for deeper self-exploration.

Your Manager Trailheads

Let's pause for a moment to give you a chance to identify some of your manager parts. Remember—a "trailhead" is any sign that helps you notice an internal part, like a tightness in your chest, a behavior, an impulse to run, a thought, a change in tone of voice, or a shift in mood.

Think of a recent event when you became overly focused on how others were reacting to you. Maybe you said something that didn't align with your true beliefs just to fit in. Or perhaps you got caught up in perfecting something to avoid criticism. Maybe you put someone down behind their back to feel superior or to create emotional distance.

Once you identify your example, play the memory back on repeat for a few moments and pay attention to how it felt emotionally and physically *at that time*. That's your trailhead! Take a moment and write down everything that you notice from this memory.

Thoughts: _____

Physical sensations: _____

Emotions: _____

Images: _____

Behaviors: _____

Anything else: _____

This trailhead can lead you to a manager part that stepped in to help. Stay with whatever you notice. You might ask the questions:

How was your reaction trying to help you?

What was it trying to protect you from?

What was it afraid might happen if you didn't think/behave/respond in this way?

If you get any answers, you have discovered a manager! This list below may help you in your journey of identifying your managers.

Common Managers

- Perfectionist (focuses on imperfections or ways things could be better)

- Inner Critic (focuses on the ways that you're not doing something well)

- Inner Judge (focuses on shoulds and should nots)

- People Pleaser (focuses on being liked by others)

- Worrywart (is unable to stop worrying)

- Fixer (tries to come up with concrete ways to resolve discomfort)

- Producer (focuses on constantly doing something)

- Actor (hides or masks feelings)

- Chameleon (changes your personality according to whom you're around)

- Controller (focuses on maintaining false sense of control)

- Blocker (builds walls around your emotions)

- Thinker (stays rational, no emotion)

- Planner (fixates on future-oriented duties or activities)

- Caretaker (focuses on other peoples' needs)

- Laundry-lister (focuses on drafting never-ending to-do lists)

Did you identify with any of the managers on that list? If so, which ones?

_____

_____

_____

_____

Learning to Do a You-Turn

You might notice a part of you saying, "It's not me—it's the things happening around me that are making me feel this way!" This is a perfect opportunity to practice a *you-turn*. Instead of blaming the people or circumstances around you for your distress, a you-turn invites you to look inward during moments of discomfort and ask yourself: *What's happening for me right now? Why am I reacting this way, and not in some other way?*

This shift in perspective creates space for *curiosity* about your experience, helping you move beyond repetitive thoughts or behaviors. By turning inward, you free yourself to respond to each situation with greater *clarity*, *creativity*, and flexibility, rather than feel stuck or trapped in old patterns.

As you begin this work, you'll start to see that often your suffering isn't caused by external events themselves, but by your internal reactions to those events. Consider this: Countless things are happening around you at any given moment that could potentially upset, distress, or worry you. So why is this specific person or experience affecting you so strongly right now? It's likely because it's triggering a memory of a past experience. In response, a part of you is reacting in the same way it did back then, repeating familiar patterns from that earlier moment.

• *Valerie's Story*

Valerie recently had a difficult interaction with a family member during a visit home. As they discussed politics, her family member expressed an opinion she disagreed with, which triggered intense anxiety. Although Valerie wanted to share her perspective, she found herself unable to speak due to the overwhelming anxiety.

Back home, Valerie felt confused about her reaction and decided to do a you-turn. She revisited the memory in detail and noticed the same anxious feelings arising in her body: Her heart raced, and she felt uncomfortably hot. As she tuned in to these sensations, she realized she was feeling scared. A voice inside her said, "Get out of there!"

Valerie was surprised by all of this going on inside and became curious about this reaction. She reflected further and was reminded of a childhood memory. She recalled overhearing her parents arguing about politics, with yelling that left her feeling the same physical anxiety and an urge to run away. These arguments were frequent in her home and had a lasting impact on her.

With this insight, Valerie felt *compassion* for the younger part of herself still affected by those experiences. As she connected with that part, her heart rate slowed, and her body relaxed. Returning to the recent interaction with her family member, she imagined calmly listening to their perspective and expressing her disagreement respectfully. This visualization helped her feel more grounded in the present as an adult, no longer trapped in her childhood dynamics. Valerie gained *confidence* in her ability to communicate effectively without fear.

Now that you've seen how this process works for someone else, let's explore some steps to help you make a you-turn!

EXERCISE: Doing a You-Turn

This is a simple technique you can do internally at any time during your day. At the start, we recommend practicing it in a quiet, distraction-free environment rather than in moments when you feel triggered or activated. As you become more comfortable and skilled with the you-turn technique, it will become easier to use it during everyday interactions.

1. Think of someone who recently upset you. It could be through their words, actions, facial expressions, or behavior. Try to bring a specific moment or situation to mind. Picture it clearly.

2. As you recall the situation, notice where you feel the upset in your body. Take a few moments to focus inward and notice your reactions.

    - Do you notice any body sensations such as tension or discomfort? If so, where do you notice that?

- What emotions are present, such as anger, fear, or sadness?

- Are there specific thoughts running through your mind? Like *They're mean. I can't stand them.* Notice any stories or judgments about the person, yourself, or the situation.

3. Consider the possibility that your reaction is coming from a part of you.

    - Is that part reacting to the current situation or is it reminded of something in your past?

    - Can you view this current situation as completely new and unique, rather than as a repeat of similar past experiences?

    - If so, what new possibilities open up for how you might respond differently to this person, situation, or challenge?

    - What internal resources or strengths become available when you choose to respond to the present moment, instead of relying on past experiences to guide your reaction?

4. If you find it difficult to see this as a new situation, that's okay. There's nothing wrong with you. This simply points to a trailhead to explore and work with the part of you that feels stuck in the past.

5. Take a moment to reflect: What was that process like, to make a you-turn and focus on your reaction rather than on the other person?

The 6 F's

The IFS model uses a helpful technique known as the 6 F's to support you in the process of getting to know an internal part. The 6 F's are a series of beautifully laid-out prompts that help you to turn inward using words that (mostly) start with the letter *f*. These words are *find*, *focus*, *flesh* out, *feel* toward, be*friend*, and *fear*:

- **Find:** Where do you find this part in or around your body?

- **Focus:** Give your full attention to the part.

- **Flesh out:** What else do you notice about it?

- **Feel toward:** Notice how you feel toward the part. Are there Self qualities present? (We ask how you feel "toward" rather than "about" to help us stay in our hearts.)

- **Befriend:** Start to build a trusting relationship with the part.

- **Fear:** Find out its fears and concerns. Provide reassurance.

Before trying to get to know a manager part with the 6 F's, start with identifying a protective part you suspect might be a manager. Reflect on your day and identify moments when your mental or emotional state noticeably shifted. For example, you might have started with a slow day at work, but when your boss gave you critical feedback, you became anxious and immediately looked for ways to be more productive. This shift—from feeling sluggish to feeling anxious—activated a productivity part. These transitions serve as valuable cues for recognizing your own manager parts. Can you recall similar moments from your day when your state changed in response to an event or situation?

Remember: The 6 F's are just for working with protectors. We will go over the process of how to work with exiles in chapter 7.

Below we'll look at an example of what it looks like to use the 6 F's to get to know a part. Then, we'll walk you through the process of getting to know your manager parts.

• *Jamie's "Grin and Bear It" Manager*

At a recent work social event, Jamie became uncomfortable when his White colleagues made comments that he found to be racist. He wanted to speak up in the moment, but something stopped him. He could feel a tug-of-war within himself—one part of him wanting to speak, while another part resisted, preferring to stay silent. He felt like running away but also felt he had to sit there and just grin and bear it.

After Jamie got home, he took some time by himself to reflect on everything that had happened. He identified this "grin and bear it" feeling as a trailhead. He decided to use the 6 F's to better understand this part.

- **Find:** *Jamie started by checking in with himself and trying to find the part somewhere in or around his body. He noticed a feeling of something behind him.*

- **Focus:** *He closed his eyes and focused on the sense of something behind him. It felt like the presence of someone standing over him with a hand on his left shoulder.*

- **Flesh out:** *As he tuned in closely, he discovered it was a shadow in the shape of a man. The shadow didn't move or have a face, but they seemed stern.*

- **Feel toward:** *Next, Jamie tried to make sense of his feelings toward that part. Initially, he wanted the part to just leave him alone, but he knew that response was likely coming from another part. It was important to Jamie to try to understand what was going on, so he asked the part that wanted the shadow part to leave him alone if they could relax and give him a little space. He noticed a sense of curiosity beginning to emerge and expressed gratitude to the part that relaxed and gave him the space to explore it.*

- **Befriend:** *Jamie asked the shadow part, "What's going on with you? Why do you have your hand on my shoulder?" The part shared that they were looking out for Jamie. The part felt it wasn't safe for Jamie to say anything in response to the racist comments. As Jamie continued to interact with this part, he learned that the part was actually young—only eleven or twelve—and they wanted to make sure he stayed quiet and safe.*

- **Fear:** *Jamie asked the part what they were afraid would happen if he spoke up about the racist comments. The part stated they were afraid Jamie would get singled out and no longer be invited to hang out with his colleagues.*

Eventually, Jamie was able to truly understand and appreciate that the "grin and bear it" part was trying to protect him. He was able to tell that part that he didn't need protection as an adult. The part relaxed and Jamie felt *compassion* for the part that stopped him from speaking up at the work event.

Now, let's have *you* give it a try. The part you choose to get to know is called the *target part*. Sometimes when we try to get to know the target part, other parts can show up. Most often we see that another part has been activated in step 4, when you ask how you are *feeling* toward the target part. If any feelings come up other than one of the eight qualities of Self (*compassion, curiosity, calm, confidence, courage, clarity, connection, creativity*), another part is present. We will guide you through how to work with that part.

Getting to Know a Manager

Before working with any internal parts, it can be important to consider your environment. Are you in a place where you feel safe and comfortable to go inside and be curious? Is the environment going to support your being able to do this internal work or will it become a distraction or trigger for other parts? Are you in a space that feels familiar and predictable or are you somewhere unfamiliar or chaotic? As you become more familiar with your internal system, it will become easier to access your parts in any environment. However, when you're starting this work, we encourage you to be intentional about choosing your surroundings.

Getting to know a part using the 6 *F*'s requires asking your part questions and listening to their responses. The following exercise gives you space to record your experience and the answers you receive from your manager parts. You can download a copy of this exercise at http://www.newharbinger.com/55909 and complete it any time you want to work with a manager. It can also be helpful to go back and complete this exercise with the same part later as you get to know it better.

When you're ready, take a moment to think about a manager (target part) you'd like to get to know. Take a few long, slow, deep breaths, allowing yourself to settle into your body. Gently close your eyes or soften your gaze toward the floor. Allow any sounds or distractions of the external world to fade into the background. As you go inside, invite qualities of your truest Self to arise in your heart. Imagine the manager you want to get to know and welcome them to be present with you. Follow the steps below:

1. **Find the part:** A part may appear as a feeling. You may hear an internal voice.

   Where do you sense the part in, on, or around your body?

   _____

   _____

   _____

What physical sensations are present, such as a tingling or tightness?

_____

_____

_____

_____

2. **Focus on the part:** Start to focus your attention more deeply. Invite any distractions to step back.

   Do the sensations or feelings in your body change at all?

   _____

   _____

   _____

3. **Flesh it out:** What else do you notice? Does the part appear as an image, thought, or feeling?

   _____

   _____

   _____

   Where are you in proximity to the part?

   _____

   _____

   _____

4. **Feel toward:** How do you *feel* toward it?

   _____

   _____

   _____

If you feel anything other than a Self quality such as *curiosity*, *compassion*, *clarity*, or *calm*, there's another part present. Take a moment to greet this part and ask if it might be able to relax and give you space to get to know your target part. You are asking the part to unblend from you. If it won't, ask what its concerns are, and acknowledge and address them. If that part can't relax, it becomes your new target part.

5.   **Befriend the part:** Once you notice enough Self-energy present (*compassion*, *curiosity*, *calmness*, or *courage*) decide how you might want to extend your care, *compassion*, concern, or *calmness* to them.

_____

_____

_____

Ask the part:

What is their job?

_____

_____

_____

How do they feel about their job?

_____

_____

_____

What part are they protecting?

_____

_____

_____

How old is this part?

_____

How old do they think you are?

_____

Can you extend appreciation for the job they are doing?

_____

_____

_____

6. **Fears:** Find out their fears and concerns. Here, we address any concerns to build trust.

   Ask the part:

   What is the part afraid would happen if they didn't do their job?

   _____

   _____

   _____

   We want to acknowledge and validate their fears. Let the part know that their fears make sense and that you understand why they are afraid.

   Then, offer some hope: "What if I could help you with your job without your worst fear happening?"

   Let the part know that you're older now and might be able to bring in a different perspective, resource, or skill that you didn't have when you were young and this part needed to take on its extreme role.

If the part dislikes their job or feels tired and weary, ask: If they were safe to step out of their role, what would they like to do instead?

_____

_____

_____

_____

_____

7. **Closing your practice session:** Before you end your practice, thank your part(s) for their willingness to communicate with you. Ask your parts if there is anything they need from you before you return to practice again.

This process of talking to your parts might feel silly or strange or disorienting at first. That's completely fine. This is a new way of interacting with yourself, and it may take time before it feels more natural. Hang in there! It will pay off in the end, we promise! (Also note: A person may do many sessions getting to know just one manager.)

A note on appreciating a part: Our protector parts work hard to keep us safe. The job is often unappreciated, and other parts in the system may dislike the protector part. That's okay. It's natural. Our job is to learn to fully understand the job the protector is doing. Why was it necessary for it to take on this role? Remember, there are no bad parts. Protectors, like managers, have a _positive intention_ even if their behavior yields negative results. Once you recognize their good intentions, you can start to appreciate their efforts and express gratitude to build a positive relationship. Here are some example phrases you might try:

- Thank you for all you do for me.

- You have a hard job.

- I appreciate how you are trying to help me.

- I see how hard you've been working.

Let's Make a Map!

We are big fans of creating *parts maps*, which are visual ways to externalize our inner landscape and to get to know and understand our parts better. It can be helpful to map out each part, whether we're working with a manager, firefighter, or exile. This is because, when we get upset about a situation, often there are many parts that get activated. It's common to have a whole posse of parts reacting! A map helps us keep track of each part we notice and helps us get the bigger picture and a better perspective on the complexities of our system.

EXERCISE: Parts Map

You can do this exercise as often as you like. A copy can be found at http://www.newharbinger. com/55909.

1. Find a quiet place where you can focus undisturbed. Once you settle in, take a few long, deep breaths.

2. In your mind, focus on a recent situation, issue, or event that was upsetting. Perhaps you had a reaction that seemed out of proportion to the event itself.

3. Write the event or issue in the center.

4. What parts can you name or identify that are reactive or upset by the event? Keep in mind a part may arise as an emotion, sensation, or thought.

5. Place a part in each circle.

6. Then, go back to each circle in orbit around the center circle. Focus on that part. Notice what the part is feeling and thinking. Write this down next to its circle.

7. Step back and take this whole picture into consideration. Most likely there's more going on than you were aware of!

8. Notice how you are feeling toward these parts. If there is a quality of Self-energy such as *calmness* or *compassion*, can you extend this quality to the part? Let each part know you hear what they are feeling and thinking. If it feels right, thank each part for trying to help you.

Great job! You now have a parts map, which gives you direction on the parts that you can explore and help. For your reference, we have included an example of a parts map in relation to a job situation.

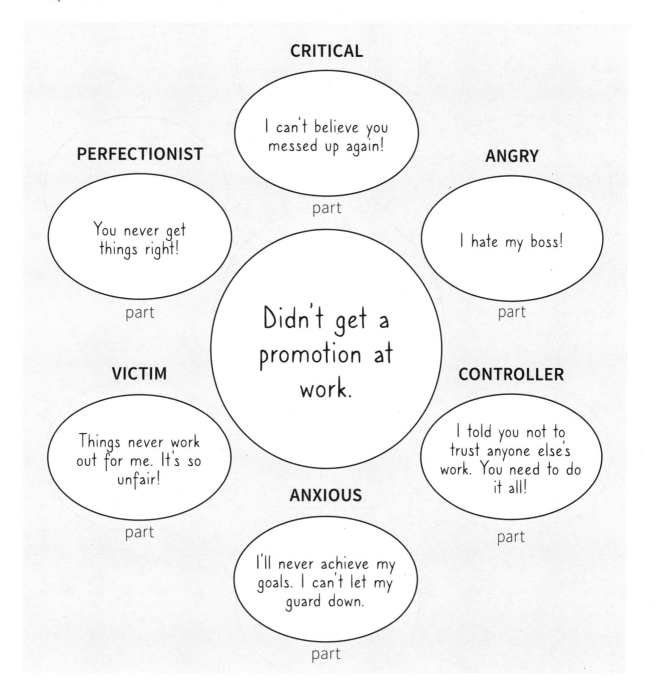

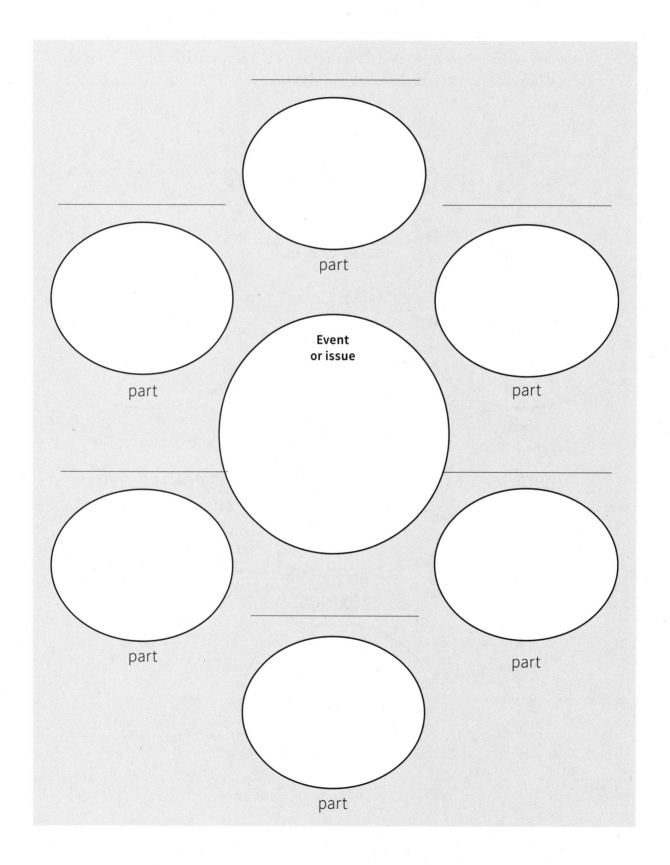

Conclusion

You're off to a great start in getting to know your manager parts! You've learned to recognize them, create space when they take over, and begin building a relationship. This is important, as managers are part of our daily lives. Understanding their intentions helps us appreciate their efforts and work collaboratively, reducing their need to blend with you and take over.

As your relationship develops and they start to trust you, you can help them unburden, update their roles, and choose for themselves how they want to operate in your internal system. For instance, a perfectionist might shift from seeking perfection to striving for excellence. Or an inner critic may decide to become a cheerleader. Remember, we're not trying to eliminate parts or make them do something against their will. With practice, you and your managers can learn to work together harmoniously. In chapter 6, we'll explore the other protector part: firefighters!

CHAPTER 6

Connecting
to Your
Firefighters

As you build your familiarity with your manager parts (and how they influence your thoughts, emotions, and behaviors), you will likely begin to notice times when you're acting or feeling not-so-managerial. For example, your perfectionist part may seek positive feedback from colleagues, but in response to criticism from a supervisor, shifts to craving and seeking alcohol or sweets. You might notice your task-focused part is absent as you spend an hour scrolling through cat videos on your phone.

What's going on? Where is that consistency and follow through that the managerial parts are often so concerned about? Perhaps your perfectionist part was working hard to protect you from feeling the sting of inadequacy only to have your supervisor's feedback do just that. If working hard fails to keep that feeling away, maybe another part will have you reaching for something else—something fun or distracting—to make you feel better.

Firefighter Parts

The above examples are depictions of how your other protector parts, firefighters, might show up in your life to try and keep you from being overwhelmed by uncomfortable or unbearable emotions coming from your vulnerable wounded parts. These parts seek to put out the "flames" of distress. Hence the name "firefighters."

Enter: The Incredible Hulk

For a sense of how these parts might show up in your internal system, it might be helpful to use a popular-culture reference to provide context.

The character of The Incredible Hulk is a mammoth green bruiser who goes on rampages and causes a lot of headaches for his alter ego, Bruce Banner. When Bruce Banner is calm and composed, he's able to go about his day. But whenever something makes his heart rate increase too much, he is suddenly overcome by an intense rage and transforms into The Hulk.

Our manager parts might have a contentious relationship with our firefighter parts just as Bruce Banner struggles with The Hulk. Our manager parts might begrudge the firefighters for carelessly coming in and wrecking all of the careful work they have done to help us fit in, keep it together, and be a productive member of society. Likewise, the firefighter parts of us might dislike how ineffective the manager parts can be at keeping away the uncomfortable or painful emotions.

Like more recent film depictions of The Hulk, the hope is that these two parts become less polarized and work together. The goal is for our internal parts to realize that the intensity of their extreme beliefs and behaviors is no longer accurate or necessary in response to the current situations that you find yourself in. Once they begin to believe this, they tend to relax and allow space for those qualities of Self (*calm, confidence, courage, creativity*) to shine through.

We all have firefighters. It's part of being human. Firefighters play an important role for us: immediate relief. They step in to keep us safe when we need distance from the vulnerability of our young wounded parts. When the emotional pain becomes unbearable, they step in to calm our psyche and nervous system. You might recognize them stepping in after you receive harsh criticism or bad news or experience something unexpected.

For Martina, one of her firefighters used to step in to bake and eat delicious cookies on cold, rainy winter days when she was down. She felt immediate relief from overwhelm. There was a calmness and boost in her mood even though she might have felt a bit icky from how many cookies she ate! Unfortunately, that was followed by guilt and embarrassment. "How could you do that? You know that many cookies are bad for your health!" stated a manager part. But the firefighter didn't care. They did their job.

Managers believe they have the best approach to keep things under control while firefighters believe their ability to react swiftly to extinguish pain is by far the more important role. There can be a bit of a problem, however. Just like a real firefighter, they rush forward to put out the fire at whatever cost necessary. They are not concerned about consequences such as broken windows or water damage to the house.

Just like in the example above, if your manager part is working hard to keep it all together at work, stay on top of responsibilities, and manage other people's expectations, they may be so exhausted by the end of the day that, once your workday is done, you feel compelled to spend the rest of your evening vegging out on the couch streaming shows on TV. That's the firefighter stepping in to give you relief. Take a moment to pause and reflect on how you tend to escape or numb out when you feel exhausted or overwhelmed and write down a few notes.

_____

_____

_____

Firefighters often get a bad rap because their extreme behaviors of numbing, yelling, or checking out are neither productive nor orderly in the eyes of the managers. Likewise, we often judge firefighters because of how reactionary they are. More accurately, other parts in our system judge the firefighters because once they step in there is no accounting for their damages. This is where inner polarizations can occur. A manager might say, "Get rid of that destructive firefighter!" and the firefighter might say, "Where was the manager when you needed them the most? I know better than that manager!" And, the more extreme the manager is, the more urgently the firefighter will try to help bring some relief, fun, excitement, novelty, you name it.

• *Mark's Story*

Mark was struggling to adjust to life as a parent. Although his daughter had been born over a year ago, he still found it challenging to navigate the changes that came with raising a child. His approach to parenting was highly task-focused. In the mornings, he concentrated on getting her up, dressed, and fed, then making sure they left the house on time so he could drop her off at daycare before heading to work. After work, his attention shifted to picking her up from daycare, feeding her dinner, and preparing her for bed.

By the end of the day, Mark was completely exhausted. Yet he felt a strong urge to stay up late, streaming shows online and drinking beer. This habit left him with poor sleep, causing him to wake up feeling terrible each morning. Frustrated with himself, Mark would criticize his behavior and vow to make better choices the next day. However, despite his promises, the same cycle repeated night after night.

As work became more demanding, Mark found himself with even less time to focus on himself. The mounting stress made him increasingly irritable with both his partner and his daughter. At times, his frustration would erupt, and he would yell in anger. Almost immediately after these outbursts, he would feel a deep sense of shame and confusion about his behavior.

To cope, Mark buried himself even deeper in work, staying late at the office and bringing tasks home. He began to resent his partner and daughter, seeing them as obstacles to his already scarce free time. This resentment led him to rush through tasks like feeding his daughter and putting her to bed, eager to crack open a beer and stream a show. However, this cycle only left him feeling more disconnected and overwhelmed.

In this example, Mark's managerial parts tried to keep him focused on tasks and productivity. The harder these parts tried, the more Mark's firefighters started showing up at home. While everyone's firefighters are unique, there are common ways these parts manifest in our emotions, thoughts, behaviors, and physical sensations. Below, we'll outline some of the firefighter behaviors that frequently show up in ourselves and our clients. Take a moment to reflect and place a check mark next to any behaviors that resonate with you:

- Rage—intense overwhelming feeling of anger or frustration

- Dissociation—feeling disconnected from your surroundings or emotions

- Numbing through use of substances (e.g., alcohol, marijuana, etc.)

- Distraction—doom scrolling, social media, binging TV shows

- Addictive behaviors—persistent desire to engage in pleasurable activities (e.g., gambling, overeating, substance use, porn)

- Any behavior that comes at the expense of other aspects of one's life, such as family, friends, physical and mental health

- Compulsive behaviors—frequent need or desire to check the news or social media

- Suicidal ideation—thoughts about ending one's life in response to stressors

- Self-harm, such as hitting, cutting, burning, or scratching oneself

- Overwhelming need or desire to sleep, rest, lie down, and so on

- Significant reduction in need or desire to sleep

- Workaholism—dedication to one's job at the expense of other aspects of one's life, such as family, friends, and physical and mental health

"I Hate My Firefighters!"

Due to the extreme nature of how firefighter parts impact our lives, it can be tempting to villainize them or wish that they would go away. After all, how can a part of you that encourages you to engage in behaviors that cause harm to yourself and others be good?

Typically, the intensity of the response from the firefighter reveals the intensity of that part's perceived threat to your survival. Perhaps a feeling of worthlessness arises after you get negative feedback from your supervisor at work. The overwhelming feeling of worthlessness can be so distressing that a firefighter part quickly steps in to extinguish the flames of emotional pain. This might lead to behaviors like overindulging in alcohol, junk food, or other substances or activities that provide temporary relief or numbness.

Notice we used the words "perceived threat." Obviously, it's not actually possible for your supervisor's feedback to kill you. However, the level of discomfort caused by that feedback might feel so intense in that moment that it can trigger the same survival instincts as if your supervisor were to pull a gun on you. From that perspective, you can imagine how some part of you might want to jump in and pull you out of harm's way.

Firefighters are incredibly selfless and deeply concerned with your well-being. The problem is that, like the manager parts, firefighters fail to recognize that you now have more control than you did during those past difficult experiences. They don't realize that as an adult, you have the ability to make choices to protect yourself from harm in ways you couldn't before. And that you can typically take care of your own basic human needs, such as food, shelter, and connection with supportive loved ones. Your survival is no longer dependent on the whims of someone bigger and older than you, so the threat to your survival is significantly diminished.

EXERCISE: Spotting Your Firefighters

As you look at the list of common firefighters, do you notice any that you can identify with? Or perhaps reading the list helped you to name your own behaviors that you can identify as firefighters trying to put out flames of pain?

Take a moment to write down your firefighter parts:

_____

_____

_____

_____

_____

As you review your notes, notice if you have any emotional reactions to those parts, such as annoyance, appreciation, frustration, shame, and write those down below.

_____

_____

_____

Think back to a recent time when you felt yourself numb out or look for a quick escape from an intense situation. Jot down a few notes:

_____

_____

Can you think of a time you raged out?

_____

_____

Can you think of a time you overindulged and then regretted it the next day?

_____

_____

Can you think of a time you suddenly and completely shut down and withdrew from a conversation?

_____

_____

When you recall that event, notice if you are judging yourself for your choices. If so, does it change the judgment if you imagine the behavior coming from your firefighter, a part in an extreme role, trying to help you?

_____

_____

Now go back through that list and see if you can identify what each part might be trying to protect you from.

_____

_____

_____

_____

_____

_____

Getting to Know a Firefighter Part

Firefighter parts typically manifest as one of two distinct and strong urges: to take action and mobilize (*hyperarousal*), or to disconnect, freeze, or shut down (*hypoarousal*). With hyperarousal, you may feel a surge of energy when reacting to a perceived threat, while with hypoarousal, you might experience a lack of or complete loss of energy to respond.

To reinforce the idea that these parts are linked to our natural survival instincts, it may be helpful to reference what we've already learned about the nervous system. In terms of the sympathetic nervous system, The Hulk wanting to smash something is a clear example of the fight response. Walking away during an argument with a friend or partner is an example of the flight response. These would both fall under the category of hyperarousal. These firefighters are highly active, meaning they drive you to take action—either moving toward or away from a perceived threat.

When those options don't result in a feeling of safety, firefighter parts will often resort to a state of immobilization, or hypoarousal, to help take you out of the moment. This response occurs in the parasympathetic nervous system and can result in dissociating, being unable to speak, or becoming intensely drowsy.

Keep in mind that the key characteristic of firefighter parts is their reactive nature. If they appear in response to something happening in the moment, rather than an attempt to prevent future harm, they are likely firefighter parts. By recognizing the pattern of reactivity, you can start identifying the firefighter parts you want to work with.

Just as with getting to know a manager part, we use the 6 F's to get to know a firefighter part. As you engage with them from a place of *curiosity, compassion,* and *calm*, these parts will begin to understand that you can handle a lot of the difficulties of your day and are capable of taking care of your exiled parts. They will start to realize that their intense concern for your survival is no longer needed at the same degree. It's through building a loving relationship with these parts that they will choose to change because they begin to trust we can take care of the wounded exiles within:

- **Find:** Where do you find this part in or around your body?

- **Focus:** Give your full attention to the part.

- **Flesh out:** What else do you notice about them?

- **Feel toward:** Notice how you feel toward the part. Are there Self qualities present such as *compassion*, *curiosity*, or *calmness*? If not, perhaps a manager part is concerned and is trying to take control (more on this in the section on tips for working with firefighters below).

- **Befriend:** Start to build a trusting relationship with the part.

- **Fear:** Find out their fears and concerns. Provide reassurance.

Before you get to know your firefighter parts, let's see how Brie applied the 6 F's to work with her firefighter.

• *Brie's Rage Firefighter*

Brie is in charge of a team of fifty and feels pressure from management above her. She works hard to keep things in order, but some days, things unravel. That's when she begins to unleash rage at her employees. Afterward she feels embarrassed and guilty. Then a people-pleaser part steps in to make everything okay, but she can tell her employees no longer trust her. She sees this cyclical pattern as a trailhead to explore using the 6 F's.

- **Find:** *Brie starts by checking in with herself and tries to find the part. She notices an intense tightness in her throat and chest.*

- **Focus:** *She gives her full attention to the sensations. It's uncomfortable and doesn't feel good, but she takes a breath and remembers to be patient and compassionate.*

- **Flesh out:** *She continues to focus and notices an image of a mean-looking man. He's glaring and shaking his fists. He seems really tense. The tightness in her chest and throat gets more intense. She takes a few long, slow, deep breaths to center herself.*

- **Feel toward:** *Next, Brie tries to understand how she feels toward the part. She wants to get the rage part under control. She feels like the part is destroying her work relationships. She notices that there's another part who wants to get the rage under control. She asks if that part can relax and give her a chance to get to know the rage part. As that part relaxes, she checks in again about how she feels toward the rage.*

   Next, she realizes she feels scared and doesn't want the rage part to be near her. After a pause, she recognizes that there is another part, a scared part. She asks the scared part if they would be able to relax and let her get to know the rage part. The scared one is a bit unsure, but says okay.

She wonders if she can bring a sense of curiosity to this rage. As she tries to do that, she senses another part is present: her controller part. This part tells her she hates the rage because they wreak havoc. She wants to get rid of the rage part, not give them more power.

She pauses to validate how the controller feels: the rage part does indeed wreak havoc. But she asks if the controller can also take a few steps back and relax. She reassures this part she isn't inviting the rage to get stronger or take control. It's been Brie's experience that when she gives a part attention, they tend to calm down, not get more powerful.

The controller finally relaxes. Brie notices she now feels genuine curiosity toward the rage.

- **Befriend:** *She asks, "What would you like me to know?" The rage part replies, "You don't appreciate me and how hard I work to keep us safe!" She lets them know that she wants to understand how raging keeps her safe.*

  The rage part is defensive. "Oh, sure. I've been helping you my entire life and now you want to get to know me?"

  Brie remembers it's important to listen and witness a part's emotions. She lets them know that she wasn't intentionally trying to avoid them and that she showed up as soon as she could. The part begins to soften a little and shares that they protect her from feeling (here she is discovering the part's positive intention).

  She invites them to share more. They say that when things get too intense, when the pressure becomes too much and she gets overwhelmed, they step in with rage to help her feel better. She begins to feel compassion toward this part as she realizes they are genuinely trying to help her. She does, in fact, feel oddly better afterward. Calmer. She expresses her appreciation.

- **Fear:** *Next, she asks the rage part what their concern would be if they didn't do their job? They say she wouldn't be able to handle it. She would go crazy or melt into a helpless puddle. She validates their concerns and asks how old she was when they first stepped in to help.*

  "Six," they say.

"Wow," she thinks to herself. "That must mean the rage part is also about six even though they seem like an angry adult!" This brings up deeper feelings of caring and compassion, which she conveys to the part. She then lets them know that she's an adult now and that she doesn't need their protection in the same way. The rage part seems surprised. She asks how they feel about their job.

"Tired," they reply.

She asks them, if she could help the part of her that feels overwhelmed and helpless, would they be interested in that? They seem doubtful, but also very interested.

Tips for Working with Firefighters

We want to pause and give some notes here because working with a firefighter can feel intense and sometimes intimidating. Keep in mind that parts can seem like they're our age, even older, but they are usually about the age of when they came in to help us.

Notice how Brie checks in to see how she feels toward the rage part several times and to check for Self-energy. If she feels one of the 8 C's, then she has enough Self presence to work with a part. If not, then she understands she is *blended* and experiencing the emotions and thoughts of another part.

When she doesn't notice Self qualities, she unblends by asking the scared part and the controller part if they can take a step back and relax so she could get to know the rage part. If either the scared or controller parts were not able to relax back, they would then become the target part. Sometimes we want to get to know a part, but if there is another part that is too concerned to relax and give us space, we then need to go to them and focus on them first.

EXERCISE: Getting to Know a Firefighter

Similar to how you track your manager parts, we encourage you to take note of each firefighter part you identify, using whatever method you prefer for keeping track of your parts. (We also encourage you to repeat this exercise using the printout at http://www.newharbinger.com/55909.) During this process, if you start to feel overwhelmed by strong emotions or sensations, take a moment to slow things down. You can do this by taking a few long, deep breaths and focusing on the feeling of your body in its present location and surroundings.

Let's begin. Take a moment to think about a firefighter (target part) you'd like to get to know. Maybe you have a specific moment you remember when you felt particularly blended with this part. Or less specifically, you are confused about how you behaved in response to someone or something.

Gently close your eyes or soften your gaze toward the floor. Allow any sounds or distractions of the external world to fade into the background. As you go inside, imagine yourself back in that exact place in time. Try to recall as many details as possible about the events that led to your awareness of this firefighter part. Where were you? Who were you with? What was happening in that exact moment when you noticed this part? What did it feel like *physically* in your body? When you feel like you're ready, follow the steps below:

1. **Find the part:** Where do you sense the part in, on, or around your body?

   What physical sensations are present, such as pressure or heat?

   _____

   _____

   _____

   Focus on the part: Start to focus your attention on the exact location of this part. Slowly move in closer. Invite any internal or external distractions to step back and make space.

   _____

   _____

   _____

2. **Flesh it out:** What else do you notice? Does the part appear as an image, thought, feeling, or sensation? Is there something specific you feel you can engage with, even if it's not entirely clear?

   _____

   _____

   _____

3. **Feel toward:** This step is especially important when working with firefighters because they tend to have strong polarizations with manager parts who want to jump in at this step to offer strong opinions. Try to distinguish between the opinions or perspectives of other parts and your own Self qualities—such as *curiosity, compassion,* or *courage*—when focusing on your target part. When you sense that enough Self-energy is present, try to imagine sending those feelings to the target part.

   Note: If you become aware of another part interfering or limiting your access to Self, take a moment to greet this part and ask if they might be able to relax and give you space to get to know your target part. If they won't, they become your new target part and you begin the 6 *F*'s with that part.

   _____

   _____

   _____

4. **Befriend the part:** Ask the part the following questions.

   What is their job?

   _____

   _____

   _____

   How do they feel about their job?

   _____

   _____

   _____

   What part are they protecting?

   _____

   _____

   _____

How old is this part?

_____

How old do they think you are?

_____

How do others react to you?

_____

_____

_____

If it feels authentic, extend appreciation to the part for the job they are doing.

_____

_____

_____

5. **Fears:** Ask the part, "What are you afraid would happen if you didn't do your job?"

_____

_____

_____

Let the part know that their fears make sense and that you understand why they are afraid. Then, offer some hope: "What if I could help you with your job without your worst fear happening?"

Let the part know that you're older now and may be able to offer a new perspective, resource, or skill that you didn't have when you were younger, at the time when this part had to take on their extreme role.

If the part dislikes their job or feels tired and weary, ask, if they were safe to step out of their role, what would they like to do instead?

Before you end your practice, thank your part(s) for their willingness to communicate with you. Ask your part if there is anything they need from you before you end your interaction with them at this time and make a note of any response they give you.

Working Retrospectively

If you're having a hard time identifying your firefighter parts or you can't seem to connect with them in the moment as easily as you can with a manager part, don't worry. This is a frequent challenge with firefighters. Because firefighter parts respond and withdraw so quickly, it can be challenging to engage with them while they are triggered. This does not mean that you are "doing it wrong" or that you "will never make any progress," which are common manager frustrations in response to trying to work with firefighters.

Instead, we recommend working with them outside of moments when you feel a direct threat, and after any immediate perceived danger has passed. Think about it this way: You wouldn't try to have a conversation with an *actual* firefighter while they were putting out a fire, would you? It's not likely that they would be open to talking with you, regardless of how *calm*, *curious*, and caring you might be at that moment. They're going to want to put out those flames ASAP!

By taking a pause with some deep, slow breaths, removing yourself from the triggering situation, or even coming back to it at another time, you will likely find it easier to engage with your firefighter parts. Then, by following the steps included in the 6 F's, these parts will begin to see that you are no longer a helpless child, that you are capable of caring for yourself, and they can dial down the intensity and even become sources of support for you as you go forward.

Relationship Repair

To address ways that firefighters might cause trouble in our personal and professional lives, we recommend making an attempt to *repair* with whomever you might have hurt or offended when blended with a firefighter part. A statement like "I'm sorry for the way that I acted and I'm taking steps to learn how to respond differently in the future" can go a long way toward reducing the collateral damage sometimes caused by these parts. Accepting responsibility for your actions can also serve as proof to any doubting parts that you are no longer a small child afraid of getting punished or ruled by feelings of embarrassment, but are instead an adult with the capacity to acknowledge mistakes and take actions to improve your behaviors.

EXERCISE: Practice a Repair

Since the practice of repairing might not come naturally or may trigger some concerned manager parts, it can be helpful to have a format to practice this technique. Use the following prompts as a guide (this will also be made available online at http://www.newharbinger.com/55909):

1. Identify actions or behaviors that caused harm that you would like to repair.

   _____

   _____

   _____

   _____

   _____

2. Identify whom you would like to repair with.

   _____

   _____

3. Pause and notice if there are any parts that might have feelings or opinions about engaging in this work and note them below.

   Part: _____ Fear: _____

   Part: _____ Fear: _____

   Part: _____ Fear: _____

   Part: _____ Fear: _____

4. Appreciate these parts' fears. See if these parts would be willing to step aside in order for you to engage in this work. If not, utilize the 6 *F*'s to work with these parts prior to attempting to repair.

5. Write out the statement you would like to make to the person or people that were impacted when you were blended with your firefighter part.

_____

_____

_____

_____

_____

_____

_____

6. Practice the statement out loud, perhaps more than once, to help you get comfortable before doing the actual repair.

Conclusion

And there you have it—your protective system! You've explored how firefighter parts show up in both your internal and external experiences and how they interact with your other protector parts, such as managers, and you've learned effective techniques to unblend from these parts. These tools will help you create a more balanced and stable internal system.

Now that you've begun to understand your system of protective parts, it's essential to keep building and strengthening your relationships with these parts before moving on to chapter 7,

"Connecting with Your Exiles." The more your protective parts feel seen, heard, and validated by the Self-led, adult version of you, the more willing they will be to step back and give you the space needed to engage with your exiled parts. This groundwork is crucial for creating the safety and trust required for the deep, transformational healing that comes from working with those exiled parts.

CHAPTER 7

Connecting with Your Exiles

As we've shared before, you already have a limitless resource for healing within you. This resource, known as "the Self," is an innate wellspring of love, *compassion*, and strength preloaded in everyone. It holds all the care and *connection* you'll ever need to nurture yourself and feel deeply in tune with those around you. You no longer need to depend on external sources for validation or healing because everything you need has been inside you all along.

Your Self—*calm, curious, courageous, confident*, and *compassionate*, has the natural ability to become the loving, nurturing inner parent that your wounded, or *exiled*, parts have been waiting for. Every step you've taken in this book so far has been preparing the way, creating the right conditions for Self to emerge and bring the love, attention, and care that your younger parts may not have received when they needed it most.

Through Self, you've already begun to cultivate a safe and loving inner world where every part of you is starting to feel seen, valued, and cared for. Now, it's time to deepen that work by exploring how Self can lovingly reach and *reparent* those exiled parts, bringing them back into *connection* and wholeness. (To access an ideal-parent meditation go to http://www.newharbinger. com/55909.)

Exiles

Exiles are parts of you that carry deep emotional pain or vulnerability from past trauma or unmet needs. These wounded parts can show up as emotional overwhelm, as intense waves of sadness, vulnerability, shame, feelings of unsafety or fear that seem disproportionate to the situation. These feelings are called *burdens* and often arise in relationship patterns: an intense fear of abandonment, sudden, inexplicable sense that intimacy is unsafe. You might also experience them as feelings of hopelessness or unexplained physical sensations. These are all potential indications of unmet needs for safely, belonging, and love.

Exiles do have the ability to release these burdens, but we will not explore the full process of *unburdening* in this book because going through all of the steps can sometimes feel overwhelming or deeply painful. As we get close to exile burdens, firefighters can step in and create backlash putting your entire system in danger.

If you feel drawn to unburdening your exiles, we warmly encourage you to do so with the guidance of a licensed IFS professional—someone who can offer safety, care, and support as you step into this tender territory. The IFS Institute (IFS-I) provides an online directory where you can find professionals trained by IFS-I: https://www.ifs-institute.com/practitioners.

What we *will* share here are the first steps in the healing journey with exiles: connection and witnessing. These steps alone can be deeply meaningful. They help you gently begin building a compassionate and trusting relationship with your exiles—a foundation for healing that grows stronger with time. While connecting with and witnessing your exiles can be profoundly healing, it is also important to understand why these parts became hidden in the first place. Exiles carry intense emotions and memories that once felt unbearable, so your system learned to push them out of awareness in order to keep you safe.

Because these feelings feel so overwhelming, they are interpreted as survival threats. To protect you from shame, terror, or grief, these parts are often "locked away"—or exiled—by protective mechanisms in your brain, psyche, and nervous system. From an evolutionary standpoint, it makes sense to push away anything that once felt life-threatening, as a way to protect ourselves from similar dangers in the future.

Exiled parts of you remain out of your conscious awareness yet carry the same intense emotional charge as the original experience. The pain of these exiles can remain close to the surface and their strong emotions can be keenly felt when triggered.

From this perspective, it's understandable why your protective parts might seem to overreact. To them, you're not just recalling a terrible event—you're *reliving* it as if it were happening in the present. They respond in the same way they did in the past because they believe that response is the best way to keep you safe; it worked for them before. Regardless of how messy or unskilled their approach is, it completes the required task of keeping you alive. Mission accomplished.

This survival-driven response reflects the deep care your protective parts have for you. Their purpose is to shield you from harm, even if their methods sometimes seem over the top. Their role isn't just to keep you physically safe—they also try to protect your heart and emotions, doing their best to shield you from emotional pain.

Recognizing a Triggered Exile

A key sign of an exile being triggered is a firefighter part stepping in to protect us. For example, when Doug's wife died unexpectedly, his deep abandonment pain surfaced, and a firefighter took over, numbing him with alcohol for months.

Exile pain can also appear as sudden emotional intensity, rawness, or vulnerability. We might want to shut down during a difficult conversation or retreat to avoid discomfort. Similarly, self-blame after a setback or deep feelings of unworthiness following rejection can signal an exile's presence.

REFLECTION: Identifying Exiles

Do any of these examples resonate with you?

Can you recall a time when you numbed yourself with food, TV, or alcohol to escape distress? Have you ever withdrawn or shut down when an old wound resurfaced? What about moments of harsh self-criticism after feeling rejected? Reflect on these patterns—could they be signals of an exile's pain? Write down any reflections:

_____

_____

_____

_____

_____

_____

_____

Why Exiles Are Banished

Remember, our manager and firefighter protectors work tirelessly to prevent us from confronting the deep pain and shame carried by our exiles.

We (Kyle and Martina) are both highly sensitive people (Aron 1996). We were given messages to "stop being so sensitive" or to "toughen up." This felt shaming and caused parts of us to feel like there was something wrong with us. As a result, our manager parts learned to give us these messages internally so we could avoid the pain of someone else making us feel bad. In this way, these protective parts hoped to provide a sense of control over how and when these negative messages came. While a highly critical part intends to help us, their harshness often reinforces feelings of inadequacy and shame rather than resolving them.

The good news is that when we start to reach our exiles, heal them, and provide our unique brand of ideal reparenting, our protectors can then begin to relax and they no longer need to engage in such extreme behaviors. Healing our exiles brings about profound emotional transformation and balance within our internal system. When we unburden our exiles, they are freed from their pain and no longer influence our lives from behind the scenes. Instead, they feel lighter, integrated, and supported. And you feel more freedom, self-acceptance, *clarity*, self-*compassion*, and *connection* to your truest Self.

Let's pause here to consider a list of common exiles. Place a check mark next to any you relate to:

I'm too much.

I'm broken.

There's something wrong with me.

I'm not lovable.

I'm not worthy.

I'm not enough.

I feel hopeless.

I feel helpless.

Everyone will abandon me.

What was that like to identify with those beliefs?

_____

_____

_____

_____

Do you carry some we haven't listed here?

_____

_____

_____

_____

Protector Fears

When you begin to access exiles, it can bring up powerful emotions. This can sometimes feel intense or even retraumatizing because exiles often carry shame and vulnerability that make them feel they may be "too much" for you to handle. But remember, you've been preparing for this—to gently sit with the discomfort of these feelings. And if it ever feels like too much, you can stop the work and take a break. And, it's absolutely okay to reach out to a professional for support.

Since a protector's job is to keep exiles deeply hidden, the main challenge in accessing an exile comes from the protectors themselves. They often block access, so it's essential to gain their permission. Building trust with protectors and addressing their concerns is a necessary step before moving forward.

Some common protector fears are:

- Protectors often worry that engaging with exiles may cause harm. For example, they may fear exiles will be seen as too needy and judged or rejected, especially if another part of you feels angry or critical toward the exile.

- Protectors also worry that strong emotions might overwhelm your system, so they work hard to keep exiles at bay.

- Since protectors don't know Self yet, they may fear exiles will re-experience their wounds instead of healing.

- They might also worry about revealing family secrets or upsetting a sense of loyalty to your family, believing you are still a child in that situation.

- Protectors often fear losing their roles or being eliminated, but they can thrive in new roles or enjoy creative freedom.

- They may also question your competence and hesitate to trust you, especially if they or the exile have felt abandoned or ignored in the past. Earning their trust requires patience, *compassion*, and consistency.

What do you recognize from the above list? What do your protectors fear?

_____

_____

_____

_____

_____

_____

_____

Because protective strategies have been in place for years, your inner system may resist change, fearing disruption, loss of control, or instability. With time, care, and trust, healing becomes possible.

I (Martina) remember my first IFS therapist talking with me about my exile that had been abandoned as a child. She said, "You've tried to manage the part that holds abandonment fear, cut it out of your life or force it to change. The one thing you haven't tried is to accept it and build a relationship with it." Those words changed my perspective. Parts of me began to relax, allowing my true Self to start connecting with and accepting that exile.

Guidelines for Gentle Interaction

Before diving in, though, we want to share some essential guidelines to help you engage with these exiles as effectively as possible:

- Be gentle, as these parts are extremely tender and susceptible to re-traumatization. Treat them as you would a hurt child, with *calm*, warm, and caring attention. If at any time you notice feelings such as fear, disgust, panic, numbness, distraction, or anything other than aspects of Self, stop what you are doing and go back to the 6 *F*'s to explore what protective part is present.

  Can you think of a child in your life that you feel warm and caring toward? How would you approach that child if they were scared or in pain?

  _____

  _____

  _____

- We cannot stress this enough: When working with exiles, you must interact with them from a place of Self. Otherwise, you are blended with a part, and you can risk retraumatizing this part of you or you may become overwhelmed, triggering a firefighter to intervene in ways that might be harmful or unsafe.

  Pause: Can you remember a time when someone treated you with warmth, *compassion*, kindness, or acceptance when you needed it most? How did it feel to receive that in that moment? What did that kind of support allow you to do?

  _____

  _____

  _____

- Slow is fast. If you experience a sense of urgency or a strong impulse to rush, it is likely coming from a protective part of you that perceives a survival threat and is attempting to act quickly to address it. This reaction is not coming from your true

Self. By slowing down, you allow yourself to access your full range of internal resources, rather than being constrained by the same limitations you faced when the trauma originally occurred.

Can you think of a time when you felt a great deal of urgency and wanted to change a situation quickly? How did that go?

_____

_____

_____

Can you recall a time when, instead of rushing, you paused and took the time to calm that sense of urgency first? How did that experience turn out?

_____

_____

_____

• Make sure the exile is safe enough to have an interaction. For example, Kyle had a client whose exiled part was actively drowning. It felt cruel to try and understand why the part was drowning _while it was drowning_, so Kyle invited the client to help this part out of the water before engaging.

Can you think of a time when you tried to interact with someone who was in distress? How did that go?

_____

_____

_____

Can you recall a time when you were interacting with someone in distress and then you became aware of their emotional state? How did you adjust your behavior after noticing their distress? How did they respond?

_____

_____

_____

_____

_____

_____

_____

_____

Asking an Exile to Not Overwhelm You

If interacting with an exile ever becomes too intense or you begin to feel a sudden wave of overwhelm, that's most likely coming from a protector part. You can always stop the exchange and revert to the regulation skills we shared earlier in this workbook. Alternatively, you can try negotiating with the part. This can be as simple as asking them to slow down and not overwhelm you. You might reassure them by saying "I truly want to understand what is happening and what you're experiencing. Can you please slow down and tell me more calmly?" Let them know that if they're screaming or flooding you with intense emotions, it will be harder for you to hear and really understand their concerns.

It does make sense that an exile might show up in this way. After all, they have been locked away and no one has come to check on them or provide support. While Self can handle any level of intensity from a part, some parts may not yet believe this. Therefore, it can be helpful to negotiate with exiled parts to share their feelings gradually, avoiding overwhelm.

EXERCISE: Engaging the Help of a Protector

For a free, reusable pdf, go to http://www.newharbinger.com/55909.

In this exercise below, we start with identifying a protector because we need to gain permission from a protector to access an exiled part. According to Richard Schwartz (2021), protectors play a vital role in our internal system by guarding our vulnerable parts—known as exiles—that carry intense emotional pain. These protective parts act as gatekeepers, and if we attempt to access an exile directly without engaging the protector, the system can react defensively, often through increased anxiety, resistance, or emotional shutdown. Instead, approaching the protector with respect and seeking its cooperation can foster a sense of internal safety and trust. When the protector recognizes that the Self is capable of managing what the exile holds, it is more likely to step back, allowing healing work with the exile to begin:

1. Engage with a protector. Identify a protector you suspect is guarding an exile. Ask the protector the following question to gain insight, and write the protector's response in the space provided (feel free to return to chapters 5 and 6 on identifying and working with protectors if needed): "What are you afraid would happen if you didn't do your job?"

   Write down the protector's response and notice the feelings or thoughts that arise. Example: The protector might say, "I'm afraid you'd feel immense pain, embarrassment, or loneliness." These emotions often reflect what the exile is experiencing.

   _____

   _____

   _____

2. Identify the exile being protected. Ask the protector: "Do you know which exiled part you are protecting?" and "Are you willing to share this with me?"

   If the answer is yes, proceed gently to step 3.

   If the answer is no, notice if the response is indirect, such as feeling distracted, spaced out, or losing focus. Stay _curious_ and nonjudgmental.

3. Seek permission to connect with the exile. Ask the protector: "May I connect with the wounded part you are guarding?"

    Notice the response:

    • A clear yes indicates permission to proceed gently. Stay present and attuned.

    • A clear or indirect no guides you to gently explore their concerns. If permission is denied, ask the protector: "What concerns do you have about me connecting with the exile?"

    _____

    _____

    _____

    _____

    How can you harness Self-energy to validate the protector's concern(s) and provide reassurance?

    _____

    _____

    _____

    _____

    _____

    Check if other protectors might have objections. For example: A protector might say, "No, we need to keep this exile hidden to stay safe."

4. Stay present and attuned:

    • If you begin to feel the emotions of the exile, stay with the experience, even if the part doesn't respond with words.

    • If permission is denied, respect the protector's boundaries and focus on addressing their concerns.

5. Avoid forcing the process. Do not force the protector to step aside. Revisit earlier steps and *continue building trust* with the protector.

6. Remember: Interacting with the exile from Self requires patience and readiness from all parts involved. Rushing can trigger strong firefighter responses. This process takes practice and patience. Honor the pace of your system as you work toward healing.

As you continue learning, remember that asking a protector for permission before approaching an exile is a vital step. This respectful interaction helps create the safety and trust needed to begin a relationship with the exile.

While we aren't exploring the full healing process of unburdening exiles here, simply taking the first steps of connecting with and witnessing an exile can be deeply meaningful. These moments of connection are powerful in themselves, and they often bring fresh movement and growth to your whole system.

Every step you take—even the smallest one—matters. By honoring the process and showing up with curiosity, care, and compassion you are already moving toward healing and transformation.

Now, it's your turn to try. Keep in mind, this process often unfolds across many sessions, so please be patient with yourself. Relationships aren't built in a day! Visit http://www.newharbinger.com/55909 for a printed and recorded version of the following exercise.

EXERCISE: Getting to Know an Exile

Connection. Where do you notice this exiled part in or around your body? How are you feeling toward this part as you prepare to engage?

_____

_____

_____

What aspects of Self are present right now? (If you are feeling anything other than one of the 8 C's, most likely you are blended with a protector part. Take time to address their concerns.)

_____

_____

_____

_____

Share with this part how you are feeling toward them (*curious, compassionate,* loving, etc.)

_____

_____

_____

How is this part responding? Are they willing to engage? For example, do they notice you are here? It's common for a part to be unsure of who you are at first. When they realize someone caring is with them, they might feel relief or even joy. However, they might also respond with anger or disappointment.

_____

_____

_____

_____

If the exiled part is not ready to engage, pause and provide a warm, nonjudgmental presence. Avoid pressuring this part to share or participate. Instead, patiently wait for them to show some willingness to engage. When you are in Self, this waiting will feel natural and unforced. If they react negatively, allow them to express their feelings and grievances freely here.

_____

_____

_____

_____

_____

If they ask questions for which you don't have answers, be honest and acknowledge that you don't know. No matter how they respond, stay present with them. To build trust and *connection*, show openness, vulnerability, and patience. Once a safe connection has been established, proceed to the next step.

Witnessing. Ask your part, "What would you like to share with me?" Wait for a response. Keep in mind that parts may not always communicate through words. They might express themselves through symbols, images, memories, or even physical sensations. What response do you notice? Write it below.

_____

_____

_____

_____

_____

_____

If you are unsure or have difficulty understanding what the part is trying to communicate, simply ask, "I'm not sure I understand. Can you tell me more or show me in a different way that I might understand?"

Write their response:

_____

_____

_____

_____

_____

_____

Remember, it's important to listen from Self and to fully empathize and validate the part's emotions and story without trying to fix or change it.

In writing, try to reflect what the part is trying to communicate to you:

_____

_____

_____

_____

_____

_____

_____

If the part shares something you deeply understand or that resonates with you, acknowledge it by expressing your understanding. For example, you might say "I *totally* get that" or "That makes sense to me."

Is there more that part would like you to know?

_____

_____

_____

_____

_____

_____

_____

_____

Building a new relationship with your exile requires ongoing care and nurturing. Make time over the next few days and weeks to check in with them. Visual reminders, like a photo of yourself as a child or a stuffed animal, can help strengthen this connection. Remember, you're building a new relationship with this part of yourself—a relationship that will grow and deepen over time

Toward Inner Harmony

As you continue your journey, it's important to emphasize that, in IFS, there is no "end goal." The work we do with our internal parts is not about unburdening every part to achieve a state where we never experience suffering again. Not only is that not possible, but approaching IFS with such an agenda is likely driven by a protective part rather than coming from a place of being Self-led.

Remember, Self does not have an agenda. The real "work" of the IFS model is to practice showing up for your parts from a place of Self again and again. Each moment of being *calm* and understanding with a part of you is an opportunity for healing. As your internal system continues to heal, it opens the door for you to extend Self-energy to others, allowing them to experience the transformative power and potential of their own Self-energy.

Conclusion

In this chapter, you have come to understand both the challenges and the beauty of working with an exile—the parts of you that hold deep pain and vulnerability. By greeting your exile with *curiosity* and *compassion*, you have taken significant steps toward building a lifelong relationship grounded in trust and care. As you continue your healing journey, you open the door to a more harmonious system led by Self.

In chapter 8, you will explore what it means to be Self-led in your relationships—whether with family, friends, colleagues, or in your roles as a parent or partner. Together, let's take a *courageous* step forward to bring more of your true Self into everyday life!

CHAPTER 8

Connecting to
Your World

Now that you've embarked on this journey of exploring your internal family system, you may see the world through fresh eyes. As your awareness of your inner parts grows, you also become more attuned to how your surroundings influence them. Have you started noticing which people and places tend to trigger your managers, firefighters, and exiles?

A manager might show up in a conversation with our partner by causing us to tune out criticism. For some, a visit with our family of origin can be deeply emotional and even painful. In these moments, our firefighters may step in to protect us, often in the form of numbing behaviors like drinking more than usual or disconnecting emotionally. Our younger, vulnerable exiles might shape significant decisions, such as selecting a romantic partner.

With so much parts-driven activity, it's no surprise that conflict can arise so easily in your relationships and surroundings. By leading from your Self instead of your parts, you can significantly enhance harmony in all your relationships. Even better, when you respond from a Self-led place, it often encourages Self-led responses from others. It's like having a superpower!

Over time, as our parts heal, release their burdens, and learn to trust the guidance of the Self, it becomes easier to lead with the Self rather than parts. This process not only increases the amount of Self-energy within us, but also creates a cumulative effect, resulting in a freer, unburdened internal system. This raises an important question: What does this shift look like in practice?

A Self-Led System

As you've been learning, parts have the remarkable ability to release their burdens and return to their original states, the way they were before taking on the roles or jobs they've been carrying. Let's delve deeper into the potential changes that can unfold when you are Self-led and these parts are freed to simply be themselves.

Managers

In chapter 5, we went over common ways that manager parts can show up in your internal system. Often focused on planning or preparing for potential threats from the external environment, managers can undergo significant shifts as these parts begin to feel appreciated and can trust in the consistency and strength of Self.

Managers that once felt they had to take over—because you were too young or vulnerable to cope—can now step back and serve as trusted advisors, supporting you as you move through daily life. For example, your inner critic might transform into an inner cheerleader, cheering you on as you go out on that first date or job interview. Your laundry lister may become like a personal assistant, helping you discern what items are important and what items can wait for another time. Once these items have been identified, your productivity part can help you kick into high gear to get things done and then stand down to make space for rest and quiet contemplation once the task has been completed.

As opposed to swooping in and taking over, these parts learn to gently tap you on the shoulder or even begin to collaborate with other parts to offer new, alternative ways of responding to daily stressors. In these ways, your parts become integrated into your complex internal system, like one big happy internal family.

When doing the IFS model, our protective parts naturally start to step out of their old roles. Think back on some of the manager parts you have built relationships with. Some of them may have simply retired and decided to take a holiday. Others may have changed and created a new role to contribute to your system positively. Below, list the managers who have changed roles. What was their previous job and what do they do now?

_____

_____

_____

_____

_____

_____

_____

_____

_____

Unburdened managers can be experienced in your internal system as:

- Creative or innovative

- Open-minded

- Efficient

- Growth oriented

- Collaborative (with other parts and people)

- Helpful or supportive

- Resourceful

- Contemplative

- *Confident*

Firefighters

In chapter 6, we explored how firefighters often step in to numb or distract you from the intense emotions of your more vulnerable parts. Just like managers, these parts can change as they recognize that you are now a capable and resourceful adult. For example, a rageful part, instead of reacting like The Incredible Hulk when upset, might transform into a source of strength and support for standing up to injustice or facing adversity. A part that once distracted you through numbing behaviors could shift into an advocate for nourishing self-care, such as meditation, creative writing, or exercise. Similarly, a part that caused sleepiness might feel re-energized and take on the role of encouraging playfulness and fun.

What was the previous job of your firefighters and what do they do now?

_____

_____

_____

_____

_____

_____

_____

Unburdened firefighters can be experienced in your internal system as:

- Responsive instead of reactive

- _Courageous_

- Energized

- Adventurous

- Spontaneous

- Passionate

- _Creative_

- Sensual

- Fun

Exiles

In chapter 7, we explored how your exiled parts carry burdens as a result of traumas or pain from your difficult experiences. Your exiled parts got locked away by your protectors to prevent the re-experiencing of those events. For example, a young part who was shamed for enjoying dance may experience a profound sense of freedom once that shame is lifted. When the impulse to dance arises, they might give in to it, finding joy and comfort in moving their body. Similarly, a young part who experienced repeated neglect from a caregiver may have come to believe they were unlovable. After unburdening, they can approach relationships with greater confidence and emotional resilience.

What would your exiles want to do if they no longer carried their burdens?

_____

_____

_____

_____

_____

_____

_____

Unburdened exiles can be experienced in your internal system as:

- Joyful

- Open-hearted

- *Curious*

- Caring

- Accepting

- Free-spirited

- Kind

- Friendly

- Innocent

- Whimsical

- Naturally wise

Your Internal and External Systems

As your parts heal and return to their true, unburdened states, this inner transformation naturally extends outward, deepening your *connections* with others. You'll find it easier to show up authentically with friends, family, and colleagues, bringing your whole self to each relationship. Old patterns that no longer serve you will start to fade, and stressful situations will feel more manageable, as the impulse to react fades away. Instead, you'll respond with *calm*, thoughtfulness, and a sense of grounded self-awareness. After moments when you're not Self-led (and trust us, there will be plenty), you'll feel more *confident* in taking responsibility for how your actions may have affected others, more *compassionate* toward parts of you that were reactive, and *clearer* about how you want to show up in the future.

Self Begets Self

In IFS we have a couple of handy phrases: "Self begets Self" and "Parts beget parts."

"Self begets Self" means that when you approach others with Self-energy, it encourages them to access their own Self-energy. For example, if you communicate calmly with a coworker using *clarity* and *compassion*, they are more likely to respond with similar qualities.

"Parts beget parts" occurs when you speak from a protective part, which can trigger similar parts in others, leading to conflict, hurt, or miscommunication. For example, if you criticize your partner, it might activate their defensive part, causing them to respond from that reactive state.

Let's try an exercise to explore how we, and others, often show up in relational interactions. This applies to all types of conversations, whether at work, in personal relationships, or with family. First, read about each style of interaction, and then try the exercise immediately after.

Self-to-Self Conversations

In these interactions, which are akin to a flow state, each person communicates from a Self-led state, showing up authentically and responding thoughtfully rather than reactively. A Self-led response acknowledges and validates the other person's feelings and concerns. For example, you might say "Thank you for sharing how you feel—I understand" or "It makes sense to me why you believe that—I appreciate your sharing your perspective." Keep in mind that Self-to-Self conversations aren't always about agreeing but about fostering respectful and constructive dialogue.

Recall a time when you felt that both you and the other person were communicating from a Self-led state.

Write down that memory: _____

_____

_____

_____

_____

Describe how that went: _____

_____

_____

_____

_____

How did it feel physically, emotionally, and mentally to feel seen and heard?

_____

_____

_____

_____

Self-to-Part Conversations

In these conversations, one person speaks from a Self-led state, while the other is blended with a part. For example, you might remain *calm* and *compassionate*, while your friend reacts from fear or anger. They are speaking directly *from a part* rather than *on behalf of* it. Approaching the interaction with Self qualities can help de-escalate the situation. When someone blended with a part receives communication from someone else in a Self-led state, they often naturally unblend and return to their own Self-led state.

Recall a time when you felt you were communicating from a Self-led state, but the other person appeared upset and seemed to be speaking from a place blended with a part.

Write down that memory: _____

_____

_____

_____

Describe what unfolded: _____

_____

_____

_____

_____

What did it feel like physically, emotionally, and mentally to listen and talk from a place of Self?

_____

_____

_____

_____

What did you observe in the other person? How did they react to your Self-energy?

_____

_____

_____

_____

It is important to keep in mind—it is not your place to name or point out someone else's parts to them. Doing so can quickly lead to conflict. Each person's journey of self-discovery is deeply personal, and even if you believe they are blended, you may be making assumptions that leave them feeling judged.

Part-to-Part Conversations

These conversations are driven by parts. Neither participant is fully grounded in their own Self-energy. This lack of stability often leads to volatility and tension, creating prime conditions for conflict and arguments to arise. These conversations can go in circles, failing to reach any resolution, and often result in hurt feelings. Neither person feels truly seen, heard, or validated, which deepens the sense of frustration and disconnection between them.

Recall a time when you had a frustrating interaction. Write down that memory:

_____

_____

_____

_____

Describe what unfolded: _____

_____

_____

_____

What were you feeling physically, emotionally, and mentally?

_____

_____

_____

_____

These reactions were likely coming from parts. Notice what parts may have been present.

_____

_____

_____

_____

Check in with those parts. Did the other person's behavior remind you of a caregiver, a previous boss, or a partner?

_____

_____

_____

_____

Can you be present with the upset parts? What do they want to share with you? What do they need from you?

_____

_____

_____

_____

Now that we've identified some common interactive patterns, it's time to explore strategies for navigating the complexities of modern relationships. One powerful perspective involves rethinking how we view challenging people, or what IFS refers to as "tor-mentors."

Tor-Mentors

Let's look deeper into our interactions with the most challenging people in our lives, who may seem like tormentors, to understand what is truly happening. When we pause and make a you-turn during interactions with perceived tormentors, we may realize that it is our internal parts reacting to the person, rather than the person causing our reaction. In the book _No Bad Parts_, Richard Schwartz (2021) suggests viewing these challenging people as "tor-_mentors_"— mentors who provide opportunities for growth, self-reflection, and healing our parts.

While it may be a tough pill to swallow, this approach can provide a way out of feeling helpless or hopeless in unavoidable familial, work, and social interactions and instead empower us to address the issue from the only place we can: the inside, out.

• *Bill and His Father*

Bill dreaded going home for the holidays due to frequent arguments with his father, which often escalated into shouting and threats to leave early. Afterward, Bill would often feel ashamed and hopeless that things would ever change.

After learning about IFS, Bill identified the parts of himself that react during these interactions. He discovered an exiled part carrying deep fear and sadness from childhood experiences with his father. By connecting with this part, Bill was able to offer the comfort they had longed for.

Next time, when his father began to raise his voice, Bill noticed the fearful part emerge. He comforted them internally, saying, "It's okay, I'm here now." Feeling calm, Bill was able to stay grounded and present, looking his father in the eyes without reacting impulsively. Instead of feeling anger, Bill felt appreciation for his father as a source of his own personal growth. Bill then expressed his love for his father and respectfully declined to engage in conversation until they could address each other with mutual respect.

Self-Led Interactions

So, how do you show up in a Self-led way? In a difficult interaction, start by recognizing when a part of you gets activated and feels hurt by the other person. Next, make a you-turn. Acknowledge and be present with that part, listening to understand why they feel upset. Then, when talking to the person who upset the part, instead of reacting from that emotional place, speak on behalf of that part—expressing its feelings *calmly* and thoughtfully.

Speaking on Behalf of a Part

Learning to speak *on behalf of* a part, rather than *from* one, helps reduce conflict, prevent hurt, and create less reactive communication. When we speak from a Self-led place, others are more likely to truly hear us—and often, they can respond from their own Self-led place as well.

Martina often uses a courtroom analogy to explain the difference between speaking directly from a part of yourself versus speaking on behalf of one. Imagine you're representing yourself in a divorce case. You're angry, exhausted, and frustrated from endless arguments with your soon-to-be ex-partner. In this emotional state, you plead your case, but your words are scattered and hard for the judge to follow. Now, imagine instead that you've hired a competent attorney. This attorney understands your perspective and knows how to present your case effectively, speaking *clearly*, *calmly*, and persuasively to the judge. Which approach do you think would yield a better outcome?

Speaking on behalf of a part might look like "When you make a comment like that, one of my parts feels deeply hurt." Or, "When you talk to me in a critical way, it triggers a defensive part of me that wants to lash out in anger." You can follow up with something like "Can we take a break and come back to talk when both of us are feeling less reactive?"

Of course, we can't be Self-led all the time; we're human. But even when we speak from a part and unintentionally hurt someone, we can still return to Self and make a meaningful, Self-led repair.

Repairing a Rupture

In close relationships, moments of disconnection—or "ruptures"—are natural and unavoidable. When someone you care about misattunes to you, it can touch tender places inside, sometimes activating wounded or protective parts. These moments can feel uncomfortable, and it's understandable to want to turn away. But when you gently tend to those parts instead, you create more safety and trust—both within yourself and in your relationships.

The first step is creating space for Self to step in and provide the attunement these parts need. We call this an internal Self-led repair, which you've already been learning to do!

But what about when we are the ones who cause a rupture?

For example, during a conversation with someone we care about, they might say something that triggers a protective, reactive, or hurt part of us. In those moments, we might yell, blame, or act in ways that damage the connection. This happens because we became blended with a part and spoke *from* them, rather than *on behalf of* them.

When this occurs, we have an opportunity to offer an external, Self-led repair. To do this, remember to first turn inward. *Connect* with the part that took over, listen to its concerns, and offer it *compassion*. From that grounded place, we can return to the relationship and repair the rupture with *courage*, *clarity*, care, and responsibility.

Think of an example from your life when you accidentally caused a hurt or rupture in a relationship with someone close to you. Write down the basic details below.

_____

_____

_____

_____

_____

Notice what parts were present when the rupture happened. List them below and how they impacted your behaviors.

_____

_____

_____

_____

_____

Take a moment to mentally rewind to just before the rupture occurred. Invite your parts to gently step back, reminding them that this is a reflection—not a real-time event. Once some space has been created, imagine yourself grounded in *calm*, *curiosity*, *compassion*, or *confidence*. Notice how this state feels in your body and how being in these qualities might have changed your response in that moment. Let the scene play out from this Self-led perspective and observe what feels different. Then, write down your reflections below.

_____

_____

_____

_____

_____

_____

Then, if it feels right, you can approach the person you had the rupture with and offer a sincere apology. This is the first step in repairing the rupture. For example, "I'm sorry for raising my voice. I wasn't angry with you. I was stressed about something else. I'll work on not taking that out on you in the future." A simple apology, even years later, can help mend a relationship.

As we practice internal repairs, our parts begin to trust that we are here for them—that we can listen, attune, and help them heal. When we extend this work outward through external repairs, we strengthen the bonds with the people we care about, and create healthier, more supportive connections in places like work.

Over time, this practice also eases the burden of needing to be perfect in our interactions, especially for parts that carry social anxiety. Our system starts to understand that relationships are not "all or nothing." Instead, they can survive missteps and grow stronger through repair — helping soften feelings of hopelessness, isolation, and fear.

When you're learning to speak on behalf of a triggered part, it can be helpful to write out a script and practice it ahead of time before having the conversation. Start by identifying a part of you that often gets triggered by that person. Remember: There are no bad parts, so be careful not to shame your parts for the jobs they have been performing.

Avoid naming or calling out others' parts. While it may be tempting to assume what's going on internally for them, this bypasses the essential you-turn—reflecting on your own experience first. Instead, share how you interpreted their words or actions, focusing on your own experience. This allows them space to recognize their own parts and take responsibility for their impact on you.

To support you in this work, we have provided a sample script below that you can use to practice being Self-led in your interactions.

EXERCISE: Write Your Self-Led Repair Script

1. Think of an upsetting or triggering situation and bring it to mind.

2. Write down how your triggered part is reacting—include their thoughts, feelings, and any physical sensations you notice in your body.

_____

_____

_____

_____

_____

3. Bring yourself into Self-energy by using the steps to work with a protector or exile. Be present with this part, listening to their concerns, pain, or shame. Let them know you see and understand them and are here to help and provide empathy, *compassion*, and reassurance. What do you want to say to this part?

_____

_____

_____

_____

_____

4. Let the part know you'll communicate with your partner, supervisor, employee, friend, or family member on their behalf. Ask the part what they want you to share.

_____

_____

_____

_____

_____

5. Imagine approaching this person when you are both calm. What would you like to say to them on behalf of this part? Remember to speak from openness and vulnerability using Self qualities such as _calmness_, _clarity_, and _compassion_.

_____

_____

_____

_____

_____

_____

Practice this script ahead of time to feel more _confident_ and grounded. Over time, as you become more present and less blended with your parts, you'll learn to speak on their behalf in the moment, even during conflict. For a pdf copy of the script, go to http://www.newharbinger.com/55909.

Being Self-Led in Romantic Relationships

Intimate relationships are hard—there's no denying that. Many of us unconsciously carry unmet needs from childhood into our adult relationships. These "young parts" of ourselves seek a sense of redemption, hoping our partner will fill the emotional gaps left by our caregivers. We hope that our partner will provide all the love, care, understanding, and attention our caregivers couldn't.

When we first meet our partner, it often feels like we are fully seen, heard, and understood—a state of perfect attunement. Early on, before our protective or wounded parts emerge, we naturally feel Self-led. It can seem like we've found someone who fulfills all we've been longing for. However, as the relationship develops, tension and conflict often arise as parts begin to surface. We may begin to feel that our partner isn't meeting our needs, or they may feel that we aren't meeting theirs. This can leave us feeling hurt and confused, wondering *Why have they changed?* We may question whether they are really "the one."

In reality, we can learn to meet our own needs. As Richard Schwartz's book *You Are the One You've Been Waiting For* (2008) explains, when you show up for yourself, your romantic relationships will be stronger for it. Understanding this dynamic can help us bring greater self-awareness and take more responsibility for our own emotional needs. Instead of relying solely on your partner to meet all your needs, think of yourself as the primary caregiver for your emotional well-being. Your partner can be seen as a secondary caregiver—someone who can support you at times but may not always be available to provide everything you need.

Self-Led with Family

For many of us, it can feel almost impossible to imagine being Self-led with family, especially if we had a challenging childhood and faced many obstacles. But we want you to know—it's absolutely possible! Family interactions can be particularly triggering for our exiles. In response, our protectors often step in to shield us, unaware that we're now capable adults. This dynamic can be further complicated by caregivers who still see us and treat us as children.

For example, Eleanor felt *confident* and successful in her daily life, but whenever her controlling father called, she would suddenly feel like a helpless child again, scrambling to justify her decisions. If he pushed her too far, her rage part would take over, leading her to yell and hang up the phone. This behavior didn't sit well with her—she was usually *calm* and *confident*. After learning IFS, Eleanor began to build a relationship with the part of her that carried rage—a part that had been protecting a deeply wounded, vulnerable exile. This exile held the pain and hurt caused by her father's controlling behavior throughout her life. As the rage part began to trust her, Eleanor was able to connect with the exile and start the process of reparenting it. With healing underway, the rage part no longer felt the need to act as a protector.

From this place of inner *connection*, Eleanor was able approach her father to make a repair. She spoke on behalf of both the rage part and the exile. She apologized for raging and expressed her need to set boundaries. She would no longer accept his controlling behavior. Ultimately, she came to understand he had his own parts and could view him through the eyes of *compassion* and *clarity*.

Keep in mind that not all family members are open to change or receptive to these types of conversations. When this happens, it's important to turn your attention inward and focus on your own growth. Even while talking to or visiting family, you can stay connected to your parts, offering them support and reassurance throughout the interaction. By doing this reparative work internally, your parts can learn to trust that you will consistently guide, care for, and love them.

Self-Led at Work

The workplace can feel like a minefield of triggers for our parts. Typically, manager parts are the ones running the show here; however, interactions with supervisors, colleagues, and employees can trigger strong and sometimes surprising reactions from our exiles and firefighters as well. Knowing how to establish and maintain boundaries in a Self-led way can support getting your needs met at work while also preventing burnout.

As you navigate setting boundaries and caring for your parts in response to work-related stress, creating a map of the parts that arise in this environment can be helpful. This map can clarify which parts respond to specific stressors, allowing you to identify those that need your support while at work and those that need support outside of work.

For example, Samira's supervisor was demanding and often overstepped professional boundaries. She frequently contacted Samira outside of work hours, insisting that tasks be completed immediately. If Samira didn't respond promptly, her boss would make passive-aggressive remarks about her work ethic. Although Samira wanted to quit, she couldn't afford to leave her job.

Using the IFS model, Samira identified two key parts affected by her supervisor's behavior: a manager part driven by financial fear, urging her "not to rock the boat," and a vulnerable part carrying a belief she wasn't good enough because of her mother shaming her in childhood. With this awareness, she approached her supervisor from a Self-led place of *courage* to advocate for clear work hours. When her request was dismissed, she remained *calm* and felt reassured by having voiced her needs. She then validated her parts' fears with *compassion*, gaining *clarity* that the job was no longer right for her and *confidence* to seek new employment opportunities.

Sometimes, supervisors or colleagues may not respect your boundaries, or workplace culture may make boundary-setting difficult. In these cases, it's crucial to care for the parts of you triggered by feelings of powerlessness or hopelessness. Take time, before or after work, to support these parts. Acknowledging and caring for them can improve your well-being and make a tough situation more bearable.

Self-Led Friendships

Friends are a true gift, often becoming our chosen family. They can offer recognition, support, and fresh perspectives that we may not always receive from relatives, partners, or colleagues. With them, we can feel truly seen and valued for who we are. Deep, meaningful friendships can also create safe spaces for healing, helping us process and mend attachment wounds from our past.

That being said, our friends have their own complex systems of parts. Even the strongest friendships face conflicts from time to time. Approaching these moments of conflict with a Self-led mindset can help mend ruptures and strengthen the bond.

Before we learn to take responsibility for our mistakes, apologizing can feel challenging. We might avoid the discomfort by pulling away, letting a friendship quietly fade—or we may find that a friend distances themself without saying why. But facing and resolving conflict, rather than avoiding it, can actually strengthen a friendship.

When we upset a friend, taking a step back with *curiosity* can help us understand what happened. Were we speaking unconsciously from a part of us, or reacting in a defensive or triggered way? Understanding our actions brings *clarity*, allowing us to sincerely repair the connection.

For example, during a conversation with his friend Sasha, Eric made a derogatory comment about Arab Americans. Offended, Sasha revealed she was of Arab descent and walked away. Overcome with shame, Eric reflected on the encounter and recognized that he had parts that had internalized prejudiced beliefs from his upbringing. He realized that the expression of these beliefs had developed as a way to seek acceptance from his caregivers and peers.

Eric later messaged Sasha, asking to meet so he could apologize. When they met, he took responsibility for his words, acknowledged their impact, and shared how the experience helped him recognize and address his biases. He committed to working on these biases so they would no longer affect Sasha or others.

What happens when we find ourself in a friendship where repeated ruptures happen, and the other person isn't able to make repairs? If we've made sincere efforts to communicate with understanding, but the other person can't meet us there, we may have to make the hard decision to let go of a friendship that no longer supports our well-being. While painful, this decision can be an important step in prioritizing our own emotional and mental health.

Self-Led Childcare

Caring for a child comes with its unique challenges. Children can often be our greatest tormentors, pushing us in ways that no other relationship does. While it's easy to focus on their "negative" behaviors and the ways they disrupt our lives, they also offer us frequent opportunities to reflect on why certain actions or behaviors trigger such strong reactions in us. In this way, children can hold a mirror up to parts of us that suffered moments of misattunement when *we* were young and provide us with the necessary trailheads to engage in deep and lasting healing of those parts. The greatest gift you can give the children in your life is a well-cared-for internal system.

As we mentioned in chapter 2, the goal of caring for a child is not to be perfectly attuned to their needs at all times. That level of attunement is not realistic, nor would it teach them how to cope with real-world challenges. This is why repairing ruptures with children is so important. When we are vulnerable and take responsibility for any harm we may have caused, whether intentional or not, we create a safe space for them. For example, you can try saying something like "I'm sorry I yelled at you. I know that hurt your feelings. I didn't sleep well last night, and when I'm really tired, I can get cranky. It's not your fault I was tired. I'll try not to yell in the future. Is there anything I can do to help you feel better?"

For additional content, such as Self-led spirituality and more on Self-led childcare, see the bonus content at http://www.newharbinger.com/55909.

Conclusion

We are excited that you have reached this point in your healing journey. Every step you take toward healing allows you to step further into your true Self, leading your life with greater *clarity*, *compassion*, and *confidence*. As you continue this work, your inner system will move toward greater harmony, creating a sense of balance and peace that extends into all areas of your life. Remember: Healing—like life—is a journey, not a destination. Each moment of growth brings you closer to wholeness. Keep going; your Self-led life is unfolding beautifully.

References

Aron, E. 1996. *The Highly Sensitive Person: How to Thrive When the World Overwhelms You.* New York: Harmony Books.

Bowlby, J. 1969, 1982. *Attachment and Loss: Vol. 1. Attachment.* New York: Basic Books.

Bretherton, I. 1992. "The Origins of Attachment Theory: John Bowlby and Mary Ainsworth." *Developmental Psychology* 28(5): 759–75.

Fogel, A. 2012. "Emotional and Physical Pain Activate Similar Brain Regions." *Psychology Today*, April 19. https://www.psychologytoday.com/us/blog/body-sense/201204/emotional-and-physical-pain-activate-similar-brain-regions.

Gitterman, D., D. MacRae, R. Kyle MacRae, and I. Parks. 2024. *Adverse Childhood Experiences (ACEs) in North Carolina, 2016–22.* Durham, NC: MDC, Inc.

Holmes, J. 2014. *John Bowlby and Attachment Theory (Makers of Modern Psychotherapy)*, 2nd ed. Oxfordshire, England: Routledge.

Howland, R. H. 2014. "Vagus Nerve Stimulation." *Current Behavioral Neuroscience Reports* 1: 64–73.

Kabat-Zinn, J. 1994. *Wherever You Go, There You Are: Mindfulness Meditation for Everyday Life.* New York: Grand Central Publishing: Hyperion.

Kabat-Zinn, J. 2013. *Full Catastrophe Living*, rev. ed. New York: Bantam Books.

McConnell, S. 2020. *Somatic Internal Family Systems Therapy: Awareness, Breath, Resonance, Movement, and Touch in Practice.* California: North Atlantic Books.

Meta Platforms, Inc., and Gallup, Inc. 2023. "The Global State of Social Connections." Washington, D.C.: Gallup, Inc. https://www.gallup.com/analytics/509675/state-of-social-connections.aspx.

Peplau, L. A., and D. Perlman. 1982. "Perspectives on Loneliness." In *Loneliness: A Sourcebook of Current Theory, Research and Therapy*, edited by L. A. Peplau and D. Perlman. New York: John Wiley & Sons.

Porges, S. 2003. "The Polyvagal Theory: Phylogenetic Contributions to Social Behavior." *Physiology & Behavior* 79(3): 503–13.

Porges, S. 2004. "Neuroception: A Subconscious System for Detecting Threats and Safety." *Zero to Three: Bulletin of the National Center for Clinical Infant Programs* 24(5): 19–24.

Porges, S. 2011. *The Polyvagal Theory: Neurophysiological Foundations of Emotions, Attachment, Communication, and Self-Regulation.* New York: W. W. Norton & Company.

Putnam, R. D. 2001. *Bowling Alone: The Collapse and Revival of American Community.* New York: Simon & Schuster.

Rogers, C. R. 1961. *On Becoming a Person: A Therapist's View of Psychotherapy.* Boston: Houghton Mifflin.

Salzberg, S. 1995. *Lovingkindness: The Revolutionary Art of Happiness.* Boston: Shambhala Publications.

Schwartz, R. 1997. *Internal Family Systems Therapy.* New York: The Guilford Press.

Schwartz, R. 2008. *You Are the One You've Been Waiting For.* Chicago: Center for Self-Leadership.

Schwartz, R. 2021. *No Bad Parts: Healing Trauma and Restoring Wholeness with the Internal Family Systems Model.* Louisville, Colorado: Sounds True Publications.

Standring, S., ed. 2015. *Gray's Anatomy: The Anatomical Basis of Clinical Practice*, 41st ed. New York: Elsevier.

Swedo, E. A., M. V. Aslam, L. L. Dahlberg, P. H. Niolon, A. S. Guinn, T. R. Simon, and J. A. Mercy. 2023. "Prevalence of Adverse Childhood Experiences Among U.S. Adults—Behavioral Risk Factor Surveillance System, 2011–2020." *Morbidity and Mortality Weekly Report* 72(26): 707–15.

Martina Williams, LCMHC, is a clinically licensed psychotherapist, coach, certified internal family systems (IFS) therapist, and consultant who has been using the IFS model since 2011. She was a trauma recovery therapist for twenty-five years, and now specializes in working with highly sensitive persons like herself. She lives in Asheville, NC, with her husband and many dogs.

Kyle Wehrend, LICSW, is a clinically licensed social worker and the owner of Move Within LLC, a private practice that provides individual and group psychotherapy, and facilitates IFS workshops and retreats. He has been working with the IFS model since 2016, and was a co-presenter at the IFS International Conference in 2023. He lives in Takoma Park, MD, with his wife, two children, and cat.

Jenna Riemersma, LPC, is a Certified IFS Therapist and IFS Clinical Consultant, author of *Altogether Us* and *IFS Integration*, and developer of the Move Toward shorthand tool for the IFS model. A seasoned clinical director and dynamic speaker, Jenna speaks to audiences across the globe, offering innovative solutions to the most challenging mental health issues of our day.

Real change *is* possible

For more than fifty years, New Harbinger has published proven-effective self-help books and pioneering workbooks to help readers of all ages and backgrounds improve mental health and well-being, and achieve lasting personal growth. In addition, our spirituality books offer profound guidance for deepening awareness and cultivating healing, self-discovery, and fulfillment.

Founded by psychologist Matthew McKay and Patrick Fanning, New Harbinger is proud to be an independent, employee-owned company. Our books reflect our core values of integrity, innovation, commitment, sustainability, compassion, and trust. Written by leaders in the field and recommended by therapists worldwide, New Harbinger books are practical, accessible, and provide real tools for real change.

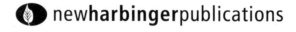 **newharbinger**publications

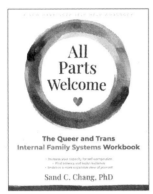
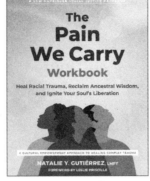
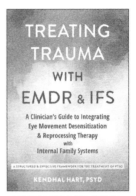
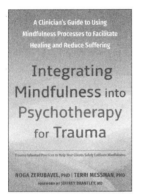
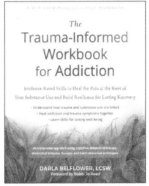
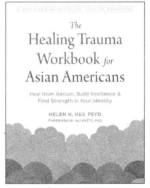

Did you know there are **free tools** you can download for this book?

Free tools are things like **worksheets**, **guided meditation exercises**, and **more** that will help you get the most out of your book.

You can download free tools for this book—whether you bought or borrowed it, in any format, from any source—from the New Harbinger website. All you need is a NewHarbinger.com account. Just use the URL provided in this book to view the free tools that are available for it. Then, click on the "download" button for the free tool you want, and follow the prompts that appear to log in to your NewHarbinger.com account and download the material.

You can also save the free tools for this book to your **Free Tools Library** so you can access them again anytime, just by logging in to your account! Just look for this button on the book's free tools page.

+ Save this to my free tools library

If you need help accessing or downloading free tools, visit **newharbinger.com/faq** or contact us at **customerservice@newharbinger.com**.